D0501221

A Recipe for Life
by the Doctor's Dietitian

Susan B. Dopart, M.S., R.D.

Co-Author and Photography **Jeffrey M. Batchelor**

Visual design and additional photography **Jessica Liu Brookshire**

A Recipe for Life by the Doctor's Dietitian

Copyright @ 2009 Susan B. Dopart and Jeffrey M. Batchelor

All rights reserved. No part of this book may be reproduced, translated, stored in a retrieval system, or transmitted, in any form or by any means, electronic, mechanical, photocopying, microfilming, recording, or otherwise, without the prior written permission of the authors, except for the inclusion of brief quotations in a review.

⊙ SGJ Publishing

Santa Monica, California

Publisher's Cataloging-In-Publication Data
(Prepared by The Donohue Group, Inc.)

Dopart, Susan B.
  A recipe for life by the doctor's dietitian / Susan B. Dopart ; co-author and photography, Jeffrey M. Batchelor ; visual design and additional photography, Jessica Liu Brookshire.

   p. : ill., charts ; cm.

  Includes bibliographical references and index.
  ISBN: 978-0-615-30873-9

1. Nutrition--Popular works. 2. Diet--Popular works. 3. Health--Popular works.
I. Batchelor, Jeffrey M. II. Brookshire, Jessica Liu. III. Title.

RA784 .D67 2009
613.2   2009907228

Dedicated to God, the Creator of Food

Contents

Foreward

I have had the privilege of working closely with Susan Dopart, M.S., R.D., throughout my 20-year career as an internist. During this time, no other physician, researcher, nurse, therapist, social worker or other health care worker has had a more profound impact on my patient population than Susan.

More patients come to my office with nutrition, weight and obesity-related problems than for any other reason. This list includes, but is not limited to: hypertension (high blood pressure), hyperlipidemia (high cholesterol), diabetes melliltus, sleep apnea, peripheral vascular disease, peripheral neuropathy, degenerative arthritis and mood disorders (depression and anxiety). These patients know there is something wrong with them as they do not feel well. And, I believe most recognize that the paths they are on will diminish both the quality and duration of their lives.

Almost all of these patients have tried and ultimately failed one dietary program after another, joined one gym or exercise-program after another, read one weight-loss book after another, tried one appetite suppressant after another, and seen one psychotherapist after another. They've traveled far and wide to weight-loss camps. They've watched talk-shows and reality-television shows dealing with weight loss. They've undergone acupuncture and hypnotherapy. Some even have resorted to liposuction and more radical and desperate bariatric procedures.

What Susan does in this book is what she does so successfully in her practice. First and foremost, she educates. What are proteins, carbohydrates and fats? What do they do and why do we need them? How do they interact with each other? What role do vitamins and minerals play in our health? What role does genetics play? What type and how long should one exercise? Understanding the answers to these questions is the first step in a nutritionally successful life. It provides the framework to which one can then add the components of what to eat, when to eat and how much to eat.

Susan also provides recipes that will please even the most discriminating gourmet, and yet they are inherently healthy and true to her message. The recipes cover all dietary preferences, and despite their extraordinary flavor, are relatively easy to prepare for those with only modest culinary skills.

Whether the reader is fit and of normal weight and desires to stay so, or unfit and overweight and in dire need of weight loss, this book will educate and empower them to make better choices for successful living and aging. I have seen this transformation in Susan's clients, including many of my own patients, over and over again. Weight loss; fitness manifested as an improvement in exercise tolerance and physical activity; the improvement or resolution of diabetes, hypertension and elevated cholesterol; rediscovering confidence in one's health and optimism in one's future health; these are all reasonable and achievable goals with Susan's guidance.

Mitchell D. Becker, M.D.

Internal Medicine, Private Practice, Santa Monica, CA
Assistant Clinical Professor of Medicine
UCLA Medical Center

Acknowledgements

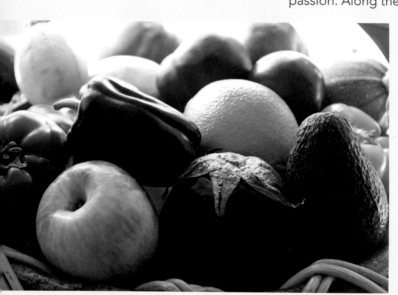

This book has been my heart's desire for many years. Helping people find happiness with food in a reasonable, healthy way has been my passion. Along the way, I have been fortunate to have been assisted by many physicians. Dr. Edwin Jacobson at UCLA Medical Center started me on the road to private practice and encouraged me to help others with what I knew. Dr. Mitchell Becker, my office partner, trusted colleague and unwavering friend, is one of the most phenomenal human beings I know. Without his tutoring, support and wisdom, I would not be who I am today.

Other physicians who helped influence me include: David Baron, M.D., Francis Dann, M.D., Albert Fuchs, M.D., Peter Galier, M.D., Tim Hayes, M.D., William Isacoff, M.D., Sheryl Ross, M.D., Timothy Schultz, D.O., Katja VanHerle, M.D., Jim Varga, M.D., and Marc Wishingrad, M.D

Other health care professionals I am grateful to include: Cindy Ahlholm, M.S., P.T., O.C.S; Steven Benedict, L.Ac., O.M.D.; Karen S. Hasler, R.N.; Christine Loeb, L.M.F.T., R.D.; Patricia McCulloch, L.Ac.; Bonnie Y. Modugno, M.S., R.D.; Barbara H. Monroe, L.M.F.T.; Polly Nelson, R.D., C.S.P.; Diana Saikali M.S., R.D.; Deborah G. Robinson, B.S., C.S.C.S., A.C.S.M; David Seals, C.P.F.T.; Anne Traynor, R.N., C.F.N.P.; Susan Weil, R.D, C.S.R.; and Ruth Ziemba, R.N., D.C.

Special thanks to those who graciously helped with hours of editing – Robin Clardy, Valerie Dillingham, Arthur Drooker, Brian Fink, and Diana Saikali. Their feedback helped bring focus and clarity to the information presented in these pages.

To the dedicated recipe testers who gave us their feedback to make the recipes easy and tasty for all to use – Jane Qualey, Brian and Jennifer Fink, Lynn Rogo, Laura Rath, Gail Block, Jeni Howland, Mitch Becker, and Jessica Liu Brookshire. To the Harris, Beckmeyer, and Qualey families, who donated props for our food photography. A special thank you to Bob's Market in Santa Monica.

To all of the clients who shared their stories, and to those wonderful clients who encouraged me for many years to write this book.

To Barbara Olivo, who helped with countless hours of recipe testing, picture taking and recipe editing. Her expertise and help was invaluable.

To Barbara H. Monroe, who spent countless hours editing for clarity and accuracy. Her assistance was invaluable.

To Melissa Balmer for her tremendous help and support with marketing and helping the book to evolve over time. Her encouragement and tutelage done with love make her advice unbeatable.

To Catherine Wire Roberts for her incredible editing skills, precision to detail and bringing friendliness to my otherwise scientific writing.

To Jessica Liu Brookshire, whose unbeatable talent is evident with the design of this book. Her countless hours of art design brought vitality to our words, and her bright, cheery disposition brought a positive force to this book.

To my parents, Joseph and Evie Dopart, and to Jeffrey's parents, Jim and Debbie Batchelor, for their encouragement to work hard and not give up on our dreams.

And last, but not least, I want to thank the most important person in my life, Jeffrey M. Batchelor, my sweetheart and partner in this life journey. Without his encouragement, insight, wisdom, and creativity, this book would not have been written. His countless hours of crafting recipes, food styling and photography brought life to each recipe in this book.

Susan B. Dopart, M.S., R.D.

Beginning Your Health Journey

Ever since I can remember, my family life was centered around food. In an Italian family, it is a sin not to have plenty of food in the house. More than double the amount of food is the norm when you have company over, and of course you always need food available if a friend arrives unexpectedly so you can play the gracious hostess!

I came from a family of great Italian cooks and bakers. But, in addition to observing how vitally important food was, I also observed health issues first-hand and faced some major challenges of my own.

My father was always hungry, and if someone was cooking or baking he was around to sample. Little did I know his hunger was related to diabetes until I was in college. Around this same time, I began having thyroid problems and ended up having surgery to remove most of my thyroid. On top of all this, I was a sophomore at U.C. Berkeley and was disenchanted with my business classes. Sitting in the hospital got me thinking – how could I avoid the health issues of my family in the future, or even better, turn that experience into something positive? Would I become diabetic like my father or other members of the family? Weight problems were already an issue on both sides, and with diabetes in my genes, the possibility of having diabetes was imminent, unless I was careful about my diet and exercise.

I found out I could get a degree at Cal in Nutrition and Clinical Dietetics, but basically had to start all over. That was okay with me. Two more years and the possibility of being more healthy over the long term seemed a fair trade off, so I jumped right in. Several years later, I found myself working as a clinical dietitian at UCLA giving traditional diet advice.

I loved helping people who were sick, but I knew my bigger mission was to help people stay out of the hospital through healthy life choices. Around that time, more studies documented how our food supply was not the safe nutritional bet it had once been. That piqued my interest in "clean eating," consuming wholesome, unprocessed food. I wanted to find ways to help others discover what clean eating could do for them.

After six years, I was ready to go into private practice with a more holistic philosophy – delving into strategies to help clients discover solutions to medical issues, emotional eating, and alternative therapies to balance their health. I explored yoga, acupuncture, and other methods to see whether they could help me or my clients.

One client I helped had weight issues after her successful battle with cancer. She dubbed me, "the Doctor's Dietitian," since her physician insisted she see me. Physicians have played, and continue to play, an important role in my career as teachers and partners, and I enjoy working with them to help our mutual clients find a better lifestyle.

As my practice grew, I had some of my own health-related issues to deal with. I realized quickly they were a blessing in disguise, intended so I might help others in a more mindful and compassionate way. My own experience has taught me that balancing food, exercise, sleep, and stress is the challenge for our society. Unfortunately, there are no easy answers, and it's up to each individual to find the solution that works best for them. This challenge becomes your recipe for life.

Therefore, the first question to ask yourself when embarking on your own lifestyle journey is, "What are my primary goals? Do I want to lose weight, improve my health, avoid or eliminate medications, improve vitality, or live longer?"

Embarking on the journey of health and balance takes time, consistency and effort. If you are willing to go the course of the journey, it can provide you with a host of rewards.

Too often, we focus on the costs of a lifestyle change. Changing that paradigm and focusing on the benefits helps make change happen.

Two key ingredients for change are *motivation* and *importance*, according to William Miller, Ph.D., and Stephen Rollnick, Ph.D., two prominent researchers in the addiction field. In their book, *Motivation Interviewing: Preparing People for Change*, they suggest that if a person has motivation, but doesn't feel the change is important, he or she will not be successful. If the change is important, but a person's motivation is lacking, alterations will not occur. The twin tenets of being motivated and deciding change is important are crucial to permanent lifestyle modifications.

Developing a lifestyle that creates a healthy weight and good health treats the cause, not the symptom. How easy it is to take medications for high blood pressure or high cholesterol to cover up an unhealthy lifestyle!

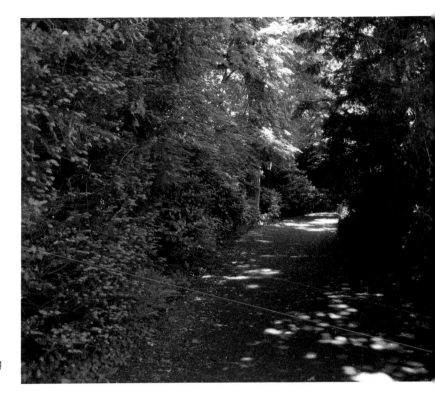

Occasionally, someone can have a healthy lifestyle, but due to genetics, needs to go on medications. Our genes determine our susceptibility to disease, but our lifestyle furthers that susceptibility. In many cases, these health concerns can be handled by changes in lifestyle. If we change our lifestyle to treat the cause of a medical issue, many times the symptoms can improve and medications can be lowered or even discontinued.

Taking charge of your health and happiness can be challenging, but the effort will provide you with rewards beyond your imagination. I invite you to join me and begin your journey to better health.

Part One

Balance is the Key: Carbohydrates, Proteins and Fats

Carbohydrate:

The First Major Player

A good first step in meeting your nutritional goals is to understand the three main components of food: carbohydrate, protein and fat. These are often referred to as the "macronutrients," since they are the major players of food. Their counterparts are the "micronutrients," things like vitamins or minerals.

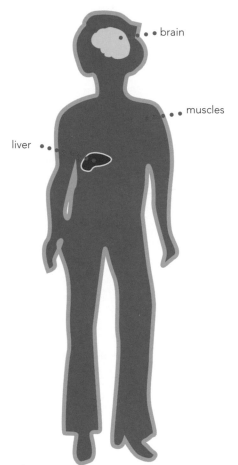

The three sites where carbohydrate is stored in the body: brain, muscles and the liver

Why is carbohydrate a major player?

- Carbohydrates are essential to life since they are needed by three major areas of the body: the brain, muscles and the liver

- Our brain needs about 80-130 grams of carbohydrate a day to maintain our blood sugar levels

If the brain does not receive what it needs, it will steal the carbohydrate from the only two other areas of the body that store carbohydrate: the liver and muscles.

Carbohydrates are measured in grams. For example, a medium-sized piece of fruit, such as an apple has about 15 grams of carbohydrate, as does a slice of bread or a cup of milk.

Let's say you are eating a piece of fruit in the morning with some cottage cheese. Since you have been fasting (not eating) during the night, your brain is saying, "feed me, feed me!" When you take the first bite of the fruit, that carbohydrate will be broken down and transported to the brain for fuel.

After your brain receives the carbohydrate it needs, the muscles are next in line, followed by the liver, where additional carbohydrate is stored for a rainy day. If you are in an active state, the carbohydrate will most likely be utilized by the muscles, which use or store carbohydrates for times of need. However, if your brain has been fed and the muscles are saturated, carbohydrate will be stored in the liver for future times when you skip a meal or decide not to eat.

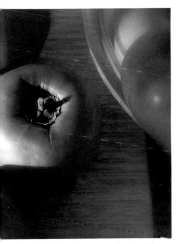

Persimmons: packed with vitamins A, C and flavonoids

When your brain or body is in need of carbohydrate, it will be released from the liver into the blood stream and go directly to the brain. If the brain does not receive the carbohydrate it needs, your body will go into a state called "ketosis."

Popular diet plans often tout ketosis as desirable, but it can lead to a breakdown of both fat and muscle to get fuel to the brain. This is problematic since muscle mass contributes to an increased metabolism, which is important in losing weight. If you are trying to lose weight, you want to keep your muscle mass in order to burn the maximum calories you can.

Losing muscle mass not only lowers your metabolism, but also means that you will need to eat fewer and fewer calories to continue losing weight – not at all my idea of a good time! This method of dieting promotes a bad cycle of changing your fat to muscle ratio. Each time you regain the weight you lost, you replace the lost muscle mass with fat.

Starved for Food

Compounding this problem, when you start eating normally, your metabolism is sluggish because you have lost large amounts of muscle mass. You start to gain weight rapidly, but now you are gaining FAT back, creating a worse situation than when you started your original diet.

This cycle is common with people who restrict their diets with very low calorie consumption or who follow low carbohydrate diets – ones that involve taking in less than 80-100 grams of carbohydrate per day. Fewer calories or low carbohydrates can mean dieters are restricting their bodies to starvation levels of nourishment. Food is a part of life; starvation is not a way of living. Eventually the body wants food. Even though such dieters may start eating normally, the weight will come back with a vengeance because they now have a compromised metabolism.

Good Carbs versus Bad Carbs?

Understanding the difference between carbohydrates is essential to learning how to eat healthfully. If you are eating food in its purest form – e.g. food which is not processed – then it's likely that you are eating a healthy form of carbohydrate.

Examples of foods that contain healthy forms of carbohydrates include:

- fruits and vegetables
- low fat plain dairy products
- nuts and seeds
- whole grains, such as brown rice and quinoa
- beans/legumes
- buckwheat

Processed and low-fiber carbohydrates include:

- pasta, potatoes, white rice

- white bread, bagels, regular or English muffins

- crackers, chips, pretzels

- most breakfast cereals

- pancakes/waffles

- ready-made desserts

Unfortunately, our culture has accepted the idea that eating grains means consuming bread, rice, pasta and potatoes in any form. These foods are low in fiber and nutrients and are essentially "filler foods."

Since the government subsidizes crops such as corn and wheat, these grains are inexpensive for food manufacturers to use in their products. As a result, consumers are faced with supermarket shelves full of processed foods that are high in calories and low in nutritional value. Imagine what would happen if the government subsidized fruits and vegetables – our nation would be much healthier.

Carbohydrates are the most quickly metabolized of the macronutrients, which means that they digest in about 1-3 hours depending on how much fiber they contain. They provide four calories per gram in addition to the many micronutrients needed for health.

The Role of Fiber

Before explaining more about carbohydrates, it's important to understand the role of fiber. There are two types of fiber, and it is easy to classify them by how they dissolve in water. **Insoluble fiber** does not dissolve in water, while **soluble fiber** dissolves partially in water.

Examples of insoluble fiber include skins of fruits, nuts and seeds, carrots, tomatoes and cucumbers. Insoluble fiber helps with creating bulk in the intestine and preventing constipation. It creates a healthy environment in the gut, lowering the risk of cancer.

Soluble fiber increases the time it takes for your stomach to digest the food, which increases fullness and creates stability with blood sugar. This is specifically helpful for those with diabetes. Examples of soluble fiber include apples, blueberries, broccoli, legumes and strawberries.

Recommended fiber guidelines for adults are between **20-35 grams** per day based on the amount of calories you take in. This is fairly easy to achieve if you are eating a non-processed, healthy diet with a lot of fruits and vegetables. Examples of fiber in fresh foods versus processed foods are as follows:,

Fiber in Foods	
Fresh Foods:	**Fiber (grams)**
1 medium apple with peel	4.37
1 medium banana	3.0
1 cup of steamed broccoli	4.68
½ cup of garbanzo beans	6.23
½ medium avocado	6.73
Processed Foods:	**Fiber (grams)**
1 medium plain bagel	1.25
1 ounce of potato chips	1.0
½ cup of cooked pasta	1.2
1 slice of pepperoni pizza	2.0
1 medium sugar cookie	.12

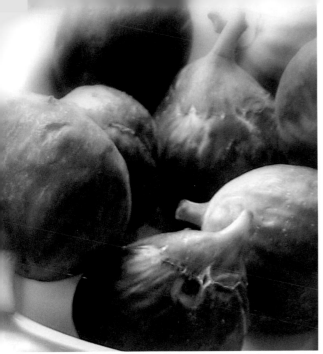

Figs: high in dietary fiber, potassium and manganese

Simple or Complex Carbs?

Carbohydrates are divided into two main categories: simple and complex. Simple carbohydrates consist of foods coming from:

- lactose - milk sugar

- fructose - fruits and vegetables

- sucrose - table sugar

Complex carbohydrates are made of a string of many simple carbohydrates of the sugar called glucose and are known as:

- Starches

- Fiber

Myth: Complex carbohydrates are the ones to focus on.

Fact: The difference between simple and complex carbohydrates is not all that significant.

Understanding Glycemic Index and Glycemic Load

David S. Ludwig, M.D., an assistant professor of pediatrics at Harvard Medical School and director of the Obesity Program at Children's Hospital in Boston, states that the "distinction between simple and complex carbohydrates has little biological significance. The most important thing is to look at the **glycemic index (GI)** and the **glycemic load (GL)**." [1]

The glycemic index is a frequently used term, but few people understand what it actually means. Basically, the GI of a food allows you to determine how high a particular food raises your blood sugar. The index is based on a number between one and 100. Examples of foods that have a *high GI* are potatoes, white rice, pasta, and white bread. Each of these has a number ranging from 65-95.

Foods with a *low GI* are whole grain carbohydrates, proteins and foods with fat. For example, nuts have a GI of 15, meaning they do not raise your blood sugar in any significant way. Sometimes we may eat one food at a time. However, most of us eat foods in **combination** like for a snack or during a meal – that's when we eat a piece of fruit and some nuts, or bread with butter. Combination meals throw the GI out the window since you would have to add up all the indexes of the foods you ate, which could end up being a complex math problem!

Walter Willett, M.D., chairman of the Nutrition Department at Harvard Medical School of Public Health, coined the term glycemic load, to indicate how much carbohydrate a person receives is based on how much of the food he or she eats.

For example, many diet books have advised against eating carrots since they have a higher GI than other vegetables. However, you would have to eat many cups of carrots to have a large GL. That's why it's important not to just look at one aspect of a food, but at the whole picture.

The GI is also dependent upon how the food comes – is it raw, boiled, fried, etc.? For example, this table illustrates the GI for carrots in two different forms:

Carrots	Raw	Peeled, boiled
Amount	⅔ cup	⅔ cup
Carbs (gms)	4.2	4.6
GI	16	41
GL	.7	1.9

As you can see, ⅔ of a cup of raw carrots has a GI of 16, whereas peeled, cooked carrots have a GI of 41. The GI of cooked carrots is higher due to less fiber (from peeling the carrot) and from the cooking process, which breaks down the cell walls. However, they both have only 4.2 and 4.6 grams of carbohydrate per serving (one third of the carbohydrates in a slice of bread.) In addition, they both have a very low GL, since there is no significant difference between .7 and 1.9. A high GL would be 50. From this example, you can see how absurd it is for diet books to recommend against eating carrots.

The GI and GL can be useful tools to someone watching what they eat, since they indicate whether a food with carbohydrate contains fiber or not.

For example, the GI of a typical slice of white bread is 70, as compared with a slice of whole wheat bread, which has a GI of 50. The white bread raises the blood sugar higher than the wheat bread since it contains very little fiber.

To take this concept a bit further, when you eat complex carbohydrates known as starches (strings of glucose molecules), it is important to choose a whole grain or whole wheat flour rather than just

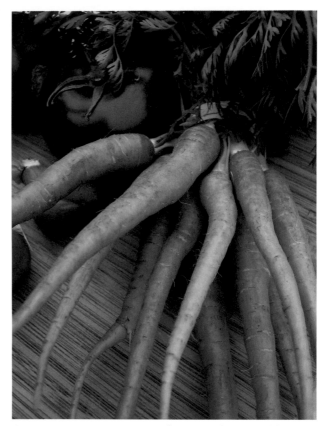

Carrots: contain over 100 types of carotenoids essential for health

wheat flour, which is processed and will not provide the same nutritional benefit. How do you know when a food is a whole grain? When reading a food label, the first ingredient needs to be "whole wheat" or "whole wheat flour."

Whole grains have a much lower GI than refined grains. As Dr. Willett states, "In our epidemiological (cause and effect) studies, we have found that a high intake of starch from refined grains and potatoes is associated with a high risk of Type 2 (adult onset) diabetes and coronary heart disease. Conversely, a greater intake of fiber is related to a lower risk of these illnesses." [2]

Looking at Carbs through a Slice of Bread:

One useful way to understand carbohydrate equivalents is to compare them to a slice of bread. For example, a slice of regular-sized bread (any type) contains approximately 15 grams of carbohydrate, which is what the American Diabetes Association uses as one serving of carbohydrate.

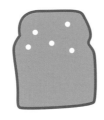

One slice of bread equals 15 grams of total carbohydrate

If you know this, you can look at any label and see how many total carbohydrates are in that particular food, or how many slices of bread's worth of carbohydrate you are consuming.

For example, the label below is for a 4-oz plain bagel. You can see it contains **61 grams** of total carbohydrate, which is equal to four slices of bread. Few people would eat four slices of bread at breakfast, but many could easily eat this size bagel.

Many times, we are not even aware that we are taking in this high an amount of carbohydrate. It's no wonder why we are gaining weight! Just reading labels for total carbohydrates is a great tool for knowing how many carbohydrates you are taking in on a regular basis. The average person needs only about 150-200 grams of carbohydrate per day unless you are an avid exerciser or an elite athlete. If you are insulin resistant (see section later in chapter) the amount would need to be adjusted to a lower level.

Nutrition Facts

Serving Size (113g)
Servings Per Container

Amount Per Serving

Calories 310	Calories from Fat 15

	% Daily Value*
Total Fat 2g	3%
Saturated Fat 0g	0%
Trans Fat --g	
Cholesterol 0mg	0%
Sodium 610mg	25%
Total Carbohydrate (61g)	20%
Dietary Fiber 3g	10%
Sugars --g	
Protein 12g	

Vitamin A 0%	•	Vitamin C 0%
Calcium 2%	•	Iron 8%

*Percent Daily Values are based on a 2,000 calorie diet. Your daily values may be higher or lower depending on your calorie needs:

	Calories:	2,000	2,500
Total Fat	Less than	65g	80g
Saturated Fat	Less than	20g	25g
Cholesterol	Less than	300mg	300mg
Sodium	Less than	2,400mg	2,400mg
Total Carbohydrate		300g	375g
Dietary Fiber		25g	30g

Calories per gram:
Fat 9 • Carbohydrate 4 • Protein 4

Beware of Hidden Sugars

Since American culture is accustomed to high levels of sweetness, many of our foods have additional sugar added. This includes anything from small yogurts to salad dressings, and many other foods you may be eating on a regular basis. The typical carton of yogurt at the grocery store has a minimum of 30 grams of carbohydrate, unless it is a plain yogurt or is sweetened with non-nutritive (i.e. artificial) sweeteners, such as Aspartame™, Sweet and Low™ or Splenda™.

Many fat-free and low fat products have sugar added, causing them to become basically high sugar products. Most juices or smoothie drinks contain 60-90 grams of carbohydrate, which would be 4-6 slices worth of bread.

The following list reveals foods that can have sugars or hidden sugars you may not be aware of:

- flavored, sweetened yogurts
- condiments, such as ketchup, barbeque or teriyaki sauce or other sauces
- any low fat or fat-free product
- salad dressings
- smoothie drinks
- canned or bottled tomato sauces
- pre-made deli case salads or entrees
- sweet relishes
- frozen vegetables and entrees
- canned fruits in syrups

- specialty waters and drinks (coffee, tea)
- processed meats

Net Carbs

A more recent gimmick introduced by food manufacturers is something called "**net carbs**," a term the food industry made up as a way to fool consumers into thinking their products contain less carbohydrates. To arrive at a net carb number, food manufacturers take carbohydrates coming from fiber or sugars known as "alcohol sugars" and subtract them from the total amount of carbohydrates.

The premise is that those carbohydrates from fiber or alcohol sugar are not processed by the body, or have minimal effects on blood sugars. Maltitol is one of the primary alcohol sugars found in foods, and it does increase blood sugar. Fiber does add bulk to food, but to think it does not add any calories or impact blood sugars is a fallacy, and has not been proven by research.

Therefore, this theory of net carbs is just folly and really only another way for food manufacturers to sell their products.

To Sweeten or Not To Sweeten?

How about non-nutritive sweeteners? There are now a variety of non-nutritive or fake sweeteners on the market, from Sweet and Low™ (saccharin), to NutraSweet™ (aspartame) to Splenda™ (sucralose). Although they are treated as substitutes, they all range from half as sweet as sugar to 8,000 times sweeter than sugar, with the average being 200-300 times sweeter than sugar.

Many diet programs and health care professionals highly advocate the use of these sweeteners, and foods containing them, to decrease the amount of sugar and calories a person takes in. What is interesting, however, is that the longer these sweeteners have been out, the more obese our nation has become. When you are consuming alternative sweeteners, you are trying to fool your body, but it doesn't work. The body **knows** what you are giving it is fake, so instead of being satisfied, it continues to give the signal that it wants to consume something sweet.

Sharon Fowler, MPH, and her colleagues at the University of Texas Health Science Center, San Antonio, collected data for eight years that was reported at the American Diabetes Association's annual meeting in San Diego in 2005. What they discovered was that people who drank diet soda did not lose weight, but gained weight. "What didn't surprise us was that total soft drink use was linked to overweight and obesity," Fowler said. "What was surprising was that when we looked at people only drinking diet soft drinks, their risk of obesity was even higher. **There was a 41 percent increase in risk of being overweight for every can or bottle of diet soft drink a person consumes each day.**"

In 2008, a study was published in the *Journal of Circulation*, which followed the health status of 9,500 men and women, ages 45-64, over a period of nine years.[3] The researchers found that the typical Western diet increased levels of metabolic syndrome (insulin resistance or carbohydrate sensitivity as described in the next section). The most surprising results of the study linked drinking a diet soda each day to a 34 percent increased risk for metabolic syndrome compared to those who drank none.

Another study done in February 2008 at Purdue University compared rats fed regular feed and yogurt sweetened with saccharin to rats that ate regular feed and yogurt sweetened with regular sugar. [4]

The rats that ate the feed and the saccharin-sweetened yogurt took in 20 percent more calories than the rats consuming regular feed and yogurt sweetened with sugar, and they gained body fat. Researchers have theorized that taking in large amounts of non-nutritive sweeteners over time conditions the body not to associate sweetness with calories, which can then disrupt the body's ability to assess caloric intake accurately and lead to overeating.

In countries where much of the food is fresh and there are less processed foods containing non-nutritive sweeteners, the multitude of low fat or "light" foods is miniscule. This may explain why the epidemic of obesity is less prevalent in countries outside the U.S. These products create the illusion that one can eat more of them and not gain weight. The body was made to process real foods that are fresh and whole, not manufactured processed foods.

Simply Resistible: Carbohydrates Gone Awry

No carbohydrate chapter would be complete without addressing the topic of **insulin resistance**.

Insulin resistance is a term that came into being in the last decade. Gerald Reaven, M.D., a professor of medicine at Stanford University, was the first scientist to identify those individuals with a conglomerate of symptoms that he coined "metabolic syndrome" or "Syndrome X."

Normally insulin, a hormone released from the pancreas, enables cells to remove glucose (sugar) from the blood stream to be used as energy. *(see diagram on page 11).* Approximately a third of the population inherits a resistance of their cells to respond properly to insulin. This results in higher circulating levels of blood glucose, which causes

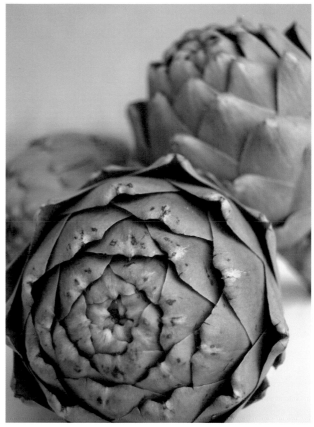

Artichokes: high in lutein for eye health

the pancreas to release ever-increasing amounts of insulin in an attempt to normalize blood glucose levels, which can eventually lead to diabetes.

Simply put, insulin is the key that unlocks the cell for sugar to get in, which in turn enables your body to use the food you consume. However, somewhere along the line, the key either gets stuck or has difficulty getting into the lock. Or, if it does get in, it cannot turn the lock, hence it was given the term "resistant." If your body develops a resistance to insulin, you are not able to utilize the food you take in, which can increase your fatigue and **cravings** for ever-increasing amounts of carbohydrate, which compounds the problem.

This resistance sets up a cascade of reactions in the body which are not in your favor. It's as if the sugar is outside the cell knocking to get in. When it cannot get in, your body keeps craving more carbohydrate. Sort of like when you eat one slice of bread - then you want the whole basket.

The pancreas, which produces your insulin, gets a signal from the body that sugar is sitting outside the cells begging to get in so the cells can feel fed. When the sugar cannot get in, the pancreas then releases more insulin. Why is this a problem? Well, increased amounts of insulin in the blood makes it easier for your body to store fat. To compound this problem, the extra sugar that is not stored as fat or used by the cells as energy goes directly to the liver. Increased levels of carbohydrate in the liver can lead to fatty liver, with the liver producing higher levels of cholesterol and triglycerides (a storage form of fat).

Insulin resistance is associated with a host of adverse health effects you'd rather avoid. This includes, but is not limited to, weight gain, high blood pressure, elevated cholesterol and triglycerides levels, diabetes, heart disease and sleep apnea.

There are varying degrees of insulin resistance with some people having a tendency and others having full-blown insulin resistance, which is adult onset diabetes. There can be a thousand-fold spectrum of insulin resistance in any one individual, meaning different levels of insulin resistance exist.

Factors contributing to insulin resistance are:

- a sedentary lifestyle

- a family history of high blood pressure, diabetes, or heart disease

- a history of gestational diabetes

- a diagnosis of high blood pressure or heart disease

- elevated triglycerides and/or low HDL-cholesterol levels

- a fasting glucose level of greater than 100 mg/dl.

The classic insulin resistant body belongs to someone who has thin arms and legs and stores much of their fat in the abdominal region. This body type is also known as apple-shaped. If you have a different type of body, or store your weight in other areas (also called pear-shaped), you may still be insulin resistant, but to a lesser degree.

In the past, insulin resistance was only seen in adults. Now, we are seeing children as young as seven-years old with insulin resistance. Research shows that one of the fastest growing populations of new onset diabetes is in teens, ages 11-17.

"Santa Claus Syndrome" (SCS), as I like to call it, can frequently happen over the holidays. You attend a holiday party and start consuming some chips, crackers, or cookies. Soon you find yourself eating a few more, and then the carbohydrate cravings go into full gear and you can't seem to stop yourself from eating. The next day you go to a holiday lunch where similar food is served. Since your body has not recovered from the night before, it keeps telling you to eat more carbohydrate. If you continue this cycle, the SCS will be in full gear, leaving you wondering how you got into this mess in the first place, or up 5 pounds during the holiday season.

Regular Metabolism of Carbohydrate

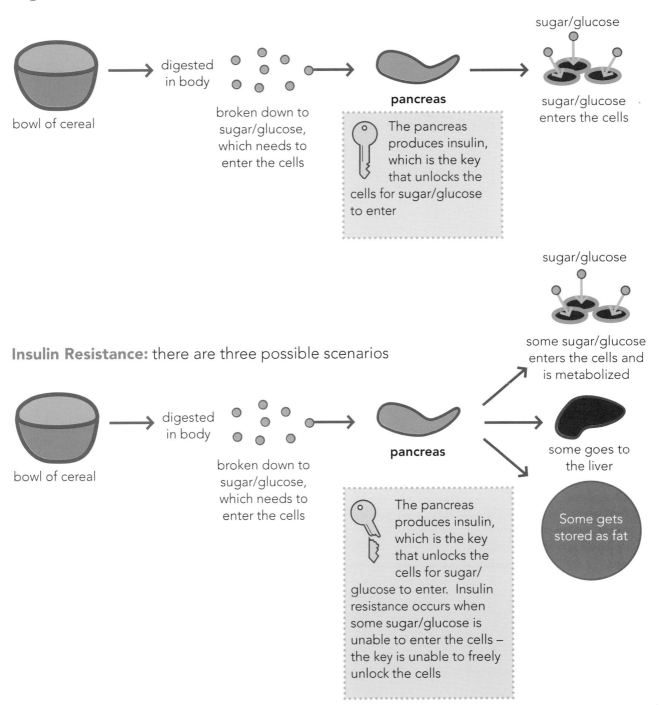

Insulin Resistance: there are three possible scenarios

Resistance is Futile:
Brian's Story

Let's take a break from the research for a moment and talk about Brian. Brian first sought nutritional guidance about six years ago on the advice of his doctor whom he saw for pain in his knees. His story clearly illustrates the symptoms of insulin resistance and how he dealt with overcoming them. Below is Brian's story in his own words.

The X-rays of my knees were negative and so was my doctor's outlook to my overall health. I was 26-years old, close to 5'6" and weighed about 214 lbs. I knew I was overweight and had struggled with weight all my life. The doctor told me all the side effects of being obese, including bad knees. I told him what he wanted to hear: "I'll try." And he told me what I needed to hear, "If you're really serious about losing weight, see a nutritionist." He then wrote down a name and number on a sheet of paper. That's how I met Susan. I knew I had to make a change and lose weight.

My first visit with Susan was truly an eye opener. My weight was high. My body fat was high. And by the time we got to my lab results, my expectations couldn't have been lower. I've had a history of high cholesterol, but never a triglyceride count that was unreadable. I was shocked and betrayed by my own body. I worked out. I played sports. I was an active person despite having an inactive job. I wanted an explanation and she gave me one. Two words, to be precise, that changed my life forever: insulin resistant.

I was tolerant of a lot of food, but not carbohydrates. I discovered my problem wasn't with inactivity. It was food. The wrong kinds of food. So we devised a plan to eat more protein and less simple processed carbs. In addition, I would monitor myself by completing a weekly food journal. My initial reaction was resistance until Susan informed me that if I didn't make a change, I would become diabetic. So, I went with the plan!

The beginning was really tough. I was hungry. I felt irritable. I was bloated. And that was only Day 1! What helped me continue was the reward she told me I would feel if I kept at it. Since whatever I was doing for the first 25 years of my life didn't seem to work, I saw this as an opportunity to make a change. I just didn't expect it to happen so fast.

In the first two weeks, I lost more than 11 pounds. Most of the loss was water, but I had some fat loss too. My diet was healthier and so was my body. I felt fewer hunger cravings and was less bloated. I began walking every day for about 30 minutes and had more energy. My body was rewarding me for eating right. However, my journey was just beginning. I still needed to clean up my diet more. No bread whatsoever, minimal alcohol and staying away from any kind of "simple" sugar foods such as desserts, candy, and sodas. I had a long way to go.

There were periods where I fell off the wagon and returned to my old habits. But doing so brought consequences. My body punished me, sometimes for days. The bloating returned, but much worse, the cravings returned, but even stronger. Again and again, I would have to "detox," but I knew I would soon feel the rewards.

It came down to finding the right balance between exercise and food. The days I ate right and exercised, my body operated like a well-tuned machine. The days I didn't, I felt "out of order." Once I stopped resisting and embraced lifestyle changes, the diet became more a part of my life and less like a diet. Instead of a medium mocha latte and croissant for breakfast, I have a bowl of low-fat cottage cheese, sliced fruit, and a few nuts on the side. Instead of a bowl of pasta and garlic bread, I have a serving of chicken or salmon and steamed vegetables. Instead of a burger and fries, I'd eat a turkey burger with no bun and a light salad. And instead of snacking on potato chips and soda, I'd have some almond butter and a little skim milk. This was a major change for me!

Now, over six years later and more than 55 pounds lighter, I feel healthier. My energy is better and most of all, I make better decisions about food. I still eat out occasionally, and every once in awhile I cheat. But during times of stress and moments of weakness when I don't feel like maintaining the diet or going to the gym, I remember my first lab results. How it felt to be bloated and most importantly those two words that changed my life: resistance is futile!

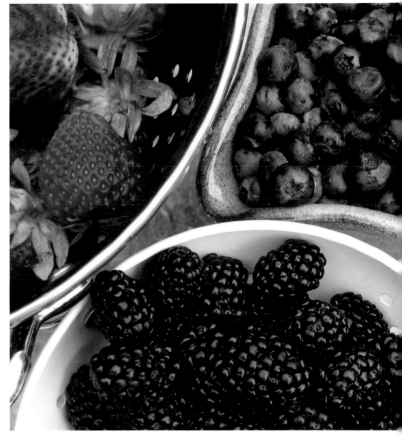

Berries: high in vitamin C, dietary fiber and manganese

Brian worked incredibly hard to change his genetics of diabetes throughout his family. He maintains his diet and exercises consistently to keep the diabetes markers in his blood under normal control.

Let's look further at how to lower insulin resistance.

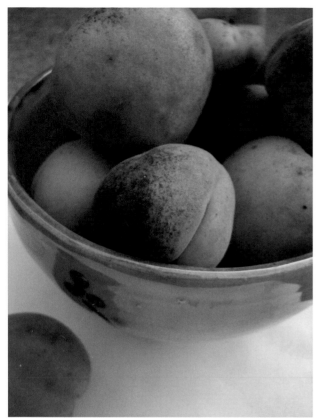

Apricots: high in vitamin A and carotenoids

The Key to Unlocking Our Cells

Since insulin is the key component to unlock the cell so sugar can get in, how can we help insulin do its job properly? One simple way is exercise. Exercise is the key to allowing insulin to work properly. In fact, daily exercise can dramatically assist in lowering insulin resistance by as much as 35-50 percent.

According to Glen Gaessar, Ph.D., a professor of kinesiology at the University of Virginia, "changing either weight or exercise patterns can have profound effects. Exercise is essential because muscle is the biggest tissue in the body – 30-40

percent of body mass is muscle. It's the major site of glucose disposal. Inactive muscle is not as sensitive to insulin." [5]

Most exercise physiologists recommend morning exercise since a person is most insulin resistant at that time. Daily morning exercise can dramatically lower insulin resistance for that day. However, exercise at any time is also very helpful. Even moderate levels of exercise (such as walking) are very powerful in lowering insulin resistance and can lead to weight loss. It is important to exercise daily since the effects usually only last for 24 hours after you exercise.

What about your diet? Diets containing moderate amounts of carbohydrate and greater amounts of protein and healthy fats at each meal can also be helpful in lowering symptoms associated with insulin resistance. Simply put:

- Start with a protein at each meal

- Add some healthy form of carbohydrate such as fruits, or veggies

- Add some healthy form of fat such as avocado or olive oil

Current research shows that simple carbohydrates coming from lactose (dairy) and natural fructose (fruits and vegetables) have less of an effect on insulin resistance and fat storage for individuals with a predisposition to insulin resistance. Starches (glucose), however, can have a greater effect.

Translation: Eating more healthy carbohydrates such as fruits, vegetables and low-fat dairy can unlock the key versus eating starchy (pasta, potatoes and white bread) and refined (chips, crackers, cookies, etc.) carbohydrates.

In 1962, James Neel, M.D., professor of human genetics at the University of Michigan Medical School, coined the term "thrifty gene." In his paper, *Diabetes Mellitus: A Thrifty Genotype Rendered Detrimental by Progress?*, Dr. Neel explained why some people gain weight and develop diabetes. [6] He wrote that individuals with insulin resistance are considered to have the thrifty gene, since their bodies hold onto weight, even in an age where there is abundance. Historically, those in developing countries with the thrifty gene survived under harsh conditions since their bodies were able to store fat easily and efficiently. In our modern world, people with the thrifty gene are at a disadvantage because they need to watch every morsel they consume. However, even if you have the thrifty gene, weight loss and maintenance are still achievable. A new regime becomes a daily endeavor with close attention paid to the type of food you are eating and to regular exercise.

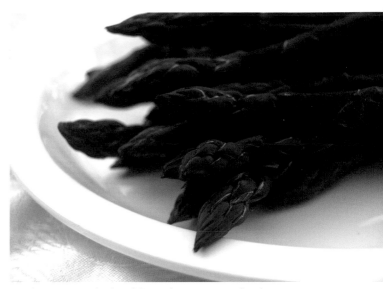

Purple asparagus: high in folic acid, vitamin K and anthocyanins

a balance of protein and healthy fats, our bodies would be in a more balanced state. When looking at the amount of carbohydrate you are taking in on a daily basis, you may be surprised at how much extra carbohydrate is in the foods you eat. Looking at the "total carbohydrate" on a label is a good way to educate yourself on how much carbohydrate the food you are consuming contains. And, beware of hidden sugars in foods like condiments, sauces and dressings.

Summary

As you can see, there is an abundance of information and research with respect to carbohydrates. The bottom line is that carbohydrates are essential for health. They provide energy, vitamins and minerals, and without them, our brains cannot function. Your genetics, your activity level, and your size all determine how much and what kind of carbohydrates you should eat.

In general, we consume many more carbohydrates than we need, and if we focused on healthier versions of unprocessed carbohydrate along with

In the chapter Balancing your Meals: Putting it all Together, you'll find information about the amounts of carbohydrate various foods contain, and how to balance your meals.

Protein:

The Second Major Player

Protein is the second player or macronutrient (major component) of food. In the same way that carbohydrates are essential to feeding our brain, protein is critical to the normal functioning of the whole body.

Protein is essential for:

- growth and repair of every cell in the body

- building muscles and bones

- making antibodies that play a role in immunity

- production of hormones

- production of red and white blood cells

- providing the nine essential amino acids needed for a healthy diet, which the body cannot make on its own

Protein takes three to four hours to digest, providing four calories per gram (the same as carbohydrate), and supplies the body with various vitamins such as B6, B12, thiamin, niacin, and minerals such as iron, selenium, zinc and copper.

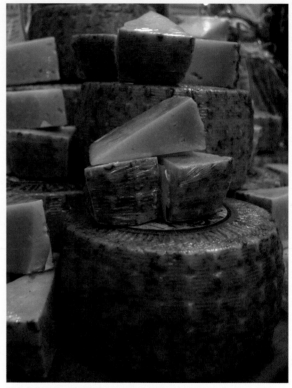
Hard cheese: high in protein and calcium

Examples of protein include:

- meat, poultry, fish
- hard cheeses, cottage or ricotta cheese
- plain yogurt, milk
- eggs
- nuts/seeds and nut butters
- beans and legumes
- natto/soybeans, tempeh, tofu

Protein is a vital part of health and well-being. Insufficient amounts of protein can leave a person feeling tired, hungry or frequently ill.

Protein is by far the most satiating of the macronutrients – that is, it helps you feel full. In the late 80's and early 90's, the "fat-free" craze was in full gear. People thought if they avoided fat they would lose weight and be healthy. They did not realize that many "fat-free" foods could actually be high carbohydrate, high calorie foods. Eating a fat-free muffin for breakfast, followed by a plate of pasta with vegetables for lunch was clearly a setup for an afternoon binge. Many individuals coming in for a consultation would say, "Something is really wrong with me – I feel like I'm addicted to food." Food addictions do exist, but many of these people simply lacked protein in their diets. Without it, they didn't have the feeling of fullness or satisfaction after eating a meal.

Jane's Journey:
From "Break-down" to Balance

Jane came in for an initial consult with the complaint that no matter what she tried she could not lose weight. I asked her to describe a typical day. This is what she revealed:

Jane was a working professional who never seemed to have enough time in the morning for breakfast. She would run off to work, stopping long enough to pick up a café latte with a non-calorie sweetener. Halfway through the morning she would feel starved. It wasn't unusual for her to seek out a bagel around the office, which she consumed with fat-free cream cheese.

Although she ate at 10 a.m., by noon she was hungry again, so she'd join her co-workers for lunch. In her attempts to be health conscious, Jane would order a salad with chicken and fat-free dressing or

dressing on the side, and a diet soda. She would try to eat only half a bread stick, but frequently ate more.

In the afternoon she would still be hungry and would find herself munching on whatever candy she could find at a co-worker's cubicle. On her way out of the office, Jane stopped at the vending machine to pick up a caffeinated diet soda, since she was tired and needed energy for the drive home.

Once at home, before changing from her work clothes, she would head straight to the refrigerator to munch on whatever was there. If a food she desired was not available, the next best option was the "death drawer" – the drawer full of processed foods that would satisfy her cravings, at least temporarily. For dinner, she would eat a balanced meal with a salad, some lean protein and vegetables. Before bed, her craving for sweets would resurface and she would give in to temptation with a bowl of cold, sugary cereal and milk. In her quest to lose weight, Jane was clearly on the wrong path.

The first thing I addressed with Jane was her lack of breakfast. Jane told me she was not hungry in the morning and only needed a coffee drink to get her energized. What was really going on was that Jane had eaten her breakfast before bed with her nightly bowl of sugary cereal and then consequently went to sleep on a full stomach.

One of the ways to solve a problem is to start at the end and work backwards, and this was the tactic I used with Jane. We discussed how she needed to go to bed a little hungry so she would be hungry in the morning upon waking or shortly thereafter. Waking up hungry is a good sign that you have not overeaten the previous day and your metabolism is healthy and ready to work. If you consume protein at breakfast such as eggs, cottage cheese, or plain yogurt with fruit and nuts it will keep you feeling full, not only in the morning, but until lunchtime. It also sets the tone for how hungry you feel later in the afternoon.

A 2008 study done at Purdue University supports this assertion about satiation and high protein foods. The study looked at overweight men who ate a normal protein breakfast (11-14 percent of calories for that meal) versus a higher protein breakfast (18-25 percent of calories for that meal). [7] The results showed the feelings of fullness were highest when the subjects consumed high-quality protein foods such as eggs, low-fat dairy or yogurt. High-quality protein refers to a food containing protein which has all the essential amino acids that the body does not make. This level of satiation was sustained throughout the day.

Translation: if you don't want to feel ravenous by lunch, eat some form of protein at breakfast such as eggs or cottage cheese. Eating cereal will leave you feeling ravenous by mid-morning because it is a low protein meal.

Jane, with reluctance, agreed to have a higher protein breakfast before she left for the office or as soon as she got to work. The next order of business was the latte with a non-calorie sweetener. In general, non-calorie sweeteners (*see Carbohydrate chapter*) can increase hunger for both food and sweet foods. Jane eventually weaned herself off the non-calorie sweetener and felt satisfied with just the latte, especially since she had her breakfast beforehand.

Since Jane was now having breakfast, the mid-morning bagel craving was not an issue. In fact, she did not even seem to notice the pastries or muffins around the office anymore. And, what about her lunch? A salad with chicken was just fine. I had her add some cheese or avocado and have olive oil and vinegar on the side. With the cheese, Jane was adding more protein and calcium. With the avocado and olive oil, Jane was adding monounsaturated and omega-3 fat sources (*see Fat chapter*).

We discussed how much protein she needed to allow her body to feel satisfied, and the amount of chicken on the salad was insufficient. Since protein is more expensive than other components of food, restaurants and eating establishments can skimp on the amount they serve you, making it necessary to add a small amount to whatever you are ordering. Since Jane felt more satisfied, the extra bread was no longer tempting, and she replaced the diet soda with a sparkling water or iced tea with lemon or lime.

carbohydrate only

carbohydrate & protein

carbohydrate, protein & fat

eat here   1   2   3   4   5   hours

Meal balance
If you eat a high-carbohydrate, low-protein breakfast, insulin levels can increase sharply, causing your blood sugar to crash within 2 - 2½ hours, stimulating hunger. If you eat a balance of protein, healthy fat, and moderate amounts of carbohydrate, insulin levels will rise more moderately, causing your blood sugars and appetite to be at a more even keel.

By mid-afternoon Jane was not craving sweets. We discussed healthy snack options, including some protein to keep her comfortable until dinner. She chose a handful of nuts and a piece of fruit. An easy tip is to bring healthy snacks to the office on Monday and then you won't have to think about snacks for the rest of the week, or be tempted by the vending machine.

On the way home, Jane was satisfied from her snack and although tired, she was fine with a bottle of water for the drive home. Once at home, she was able to change her work clothes and start making dinner for herself and her family. The "death drawer" no longer existed and the refrigerator was filled with fruit, cut-up veggies, string cheese, natural peanut butter and other healthy snacks if she needed or craved something prior to dinner. After dinner, she wanted a little something sweet for enjoyment, so we added good-quality dark chocolate. She found herself satisfied with a square or two and a cup of tea. Jane decided not to eat after 8 p.m. to ensure waking up with a healthy hunger.

In about six weeks, all the changes Jane incorporated into her diet caused her to feel more energized throughout the day. Because she no longer was starved or ravenous, she was able to regulate her food. In the following months, she lost the weight she was determined to shed.

Protein and Hunger

Having enough protein in your diet is **critical** for many reasons, including regulating your appetite. "Having some sort of protein at each meal and snack can increase satiation and literally turn off the hunger mechanism in your head," says Rick Mattes, Ph.D., M.P.H., R.D., a researcher in the Department of Foods and Nutrition at Purdue University. Dr. Mattes, who has done multiple research studies on

what increases satiation in the diet, stresses that protein has the strongest satiety value, meaning no other macronutrient can make you feel as full as protein. [8]

Besides making you feel full, eating protein can decrease your appetite. In 2006, Rachel Batterham, Ph.D., and researchers at the University College of London, conducted studies showing that when subjects ate protein (versus carbohydrate or fat) their stomachs secreted hormones that lowered their appetites. [9] The subjects ate one-third less calories than they normally consumed.

Ghrelin and Leptin
To really understand what's behind feeling hungry or full, it's worth knowing a bit about two hormones – *ghrelin* (pronounced gar-elin) and *leptin*. Researchers are just beginning to understand the full significance of these hormones on our appetites.

In 2007, David Cummings, M.D., and colleagues at the University School of Medicine in Seattle, published multiple studies on *ghrelin*, a hormone that can increase body weight since it stimulates the appetite.[10] Ghrelin can be affected by what you eat and how much you sleep. Understanding how ghrelin works in the body is important since it correlates highly with food intake.

In contrast to ghrelin, which makes you feel hungry, leptin is the hormone that causes you to feel full. These hormones work to your advantage when your diet is in balance and you are receiving adequate rest, and to your detriment when your diet is out of balance and you are lacking sleep. An easy way to think about it is that **ghrelin grows your appetite and leptin lowers it**. The macronutrients (carbohydrate, protein and fat) you eat affect these hormones.

	Ghrelin Levels	Hunger Levels
Carbohydrate	briefly decrease, then increase sharply	increase sharply
Protein	decreased	decreased
Fat	neutral	neutral

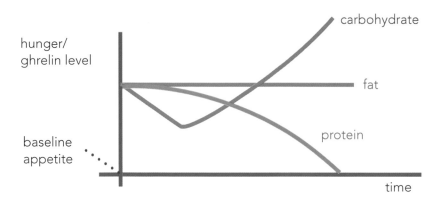

carbohydrate initially drops hunger levels, and then hunger rebounds up

protein lowers hunger levels

fat has a neutral effect on hunger levels

Dr. Cummings found that proteins were the best suppressors of appetite. Fats seemed to have a neutral effect on appetite. Carbohydrates initially lowered the appetite, but then rebounded soon afterward with a vengeance – causing the appetite to be even greater than before the food was introduced. The above chart summarizes the findings of this research.

Protein and Your Metabolism

When people speak about metabolism, what exactly do they mean? Basically, metabolism is the rate at which your body burns calories.

A review in *Clinical Nutrition and Metabolic Care* (2003) states that consuming more protein can induce a higher metabolism or thermogenesis (production of heat by the body), and a higher level of fullness after eating. [11]

If you want to burn more calories and keep your metabolism strong, consume regular amounts of protein at meals and snacks.

A 2002 study published in the *Journal of the American College of Nutrition* tested the number of calories burned when subjects consumed a high-protein, low-fat diet versus a high-carbohydrate, low-fat diet.[12] An example of these meal comparisons would be having a chicken breast with some vegetables, versus having some pasta with vegetables. **Individuals consuming the higher protein diet had metabolisms registering two times higher 2.5 hours after their meals than those consuming the high-carbohydrate diet.** This finding could explain why people consuming more protein lose weight.

How much protein do you actually need?

Multiple research articles exist that give differing opinions from nutritionists and doctors on how much protein we really need. When figuring out protein needs, it is essential to look at the needs of the individual. Protein needs are affected by:

- your sex and age

- how much exercise and/or activity you get during the course of the week

- specific medical problems that would dictate how much protein you need or are allowed

Therefore, one generic protein recommendation does not fit all. In general, estimated protein needs are based on an individual's weight, age, exercise level and medical needs.

Most dietetic associations and organizations recommend the RDA (Recommended Daily Allowance) of .8-1.0 grams of protein per kilogram (2.2 pounds) body weight per day. In practice and theory, this amount is at the lower level that a sedentary person would require. Active, exercising people need more protein than the RDA. Studies show that an active individual needs at least 1.3-1.5 grams of protein per kilogram of body weight. How do we translate this into understandable terms?

Let's take Bill, a 45-year-old, 180-pound male who is generally healthy, has a normal weight for his height, and exercises a of couple times a week by walking and going to the gym.

- Bill is 180 pounds (or 180 divided by 2.2 =81.8 kilograms)

- 81.8 kilograms x 1.3 to 1.5 grams of protein per kg = 106 to 123 grams of protein per day

Bill could easily meet the majority of his protein needs with 1 cup of cottage cheese for breakfast (32 grams of protein), a lean 5-ounce hamburger at lunch (35 grams) and a salmon filet at dinner (about 5 ounces or 35 grams of protein). The rest of the food in his meals would easily make up the balance of his protein requirements.

Average Adult Needs for Protein

What about the average adult? If you are active or have some sort of exercise regimen such as light walking, 20-30 minutes several times per week, your protein needs increase to at least 1.1 to 1.3 grams per kilogram. If you are more athletic, the amount could increase to 1.5 to 2.0 grams per kilogram.

So, how does this translate into real eating?

- If you are 140 pounds (or approximately 64 kilograms) and are sedentary, you would need about 55 to 65 grams (.8-1 gm/kg body weight) of protein per day.

- If you are more active and/or walk or exercise several times per week, then you would need about 80-95 (1.1 to 1.3 gm/kg body weight) grams of protein.

- If you work out 5-6 days per week at higher intensities, you would need about 100-130 (1.5 to 2 gm/kg body weight) grams of protein.

Later chapters will outline how to translate these amounts into practical eating.

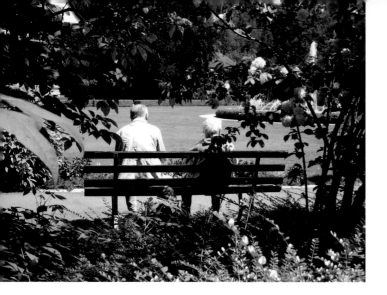

Older Adults

Another thing to be aware of is that protein needs increase as we age. William J. Evans, Ph.D., the director of the Nutrition, Metabolism, and Exercise Laboratory at the University of Arkansas for Medical Sciences, has done extensive research on protein needs, both in athletes and older adults. His findings indicate that as we age our protein needs rise, even if we do not exercise. Studies done by Dr. Evans indicate that physically inactive adults who ate the RDA (.8 grams/kg) for protein for a period of four months lost muscle mass.[13]

Dr. Evans studied older adults who ate the RDA for protein, but added weight-training three times per week. The amount of protein was still inadequate for muscle maintenance, but the weight training helped preserve the muscle against some loss.[14] The study concluded that if the subjects doubled their protein intake to 1.6 grams of protein per kilogram and added weight/strength training to their regimen, that was the best of both possible worlds: protein needs were met and muscle mass was maintained or increased. Most studies done on geriatric adults (over age 70) indicate that they do not process protein as well, and as they age they require approximately 1.4 grams of protein per kilogram to maintain their muscle mass or integrity.

High Protein Diets: Myths versus Facts

As important as the research indicates protein to be, much criticism exists regarding high protein diets. Eating protein at each meal and snack does not necessarily translate to a "high protein" diet. There is a vast difference between consuming regular amounts of protein and "high protein."

Let's look at some of the myths around protein.

Myth: Protein can damage kidneys.

Fact: Articles have been circulated through the years stating that protein in the diet can damage the kidneys, but studies conducted on people consuming varying levels of protein do not show that restricting protein prevents decline in kidney function. In 2004, an article published in *Sports Nutrition Review Journal* supported this, stating:

> *"Despite its role in nitrogen excretion (that is, getting rid of the waste products of protein ingested), there are presently no data in the scientific literature demonstrating that a healthy kidney will be damaged by increased demands of protein consumed above the Recommended Dietary Allowance (RDA). Furthermore, real world examples support this contention, since kidney issues are nonexistent in the body building community in which high-protein intake has been the norm for over half a century."*[15]

Translation: There is no reason to restrict protein in individuals with healthy kidneys.

Myth: Diets with higher protein are dangerous to bone health.

Fact: Research in the last few years found the opposite to be true. Recent studies show lower amounts of protein in the diet can be associated with bone loss, especially in older individuals. Bess Dawson-Hughes, M.D., wrote a review on studies done at the U.S. Department of Agriculture Human Nutrition Research Center on Aging at Tufts University. Dr. Dawson-Hughes found adequate protein intake significantly reduced bone loss in elderly hip-fracture patients, and that bone loss was even less when the subjects received supplemental calcium.[16]

Myth: Protein is bad for diabetics.

Fact: With respect to protein and its effect on blood sugars, Mary C. Gannon, Ph.D., at the Metabolic Research Laboratory and the Section of Endocrinology, Metabolism, and Nutrition at the Department of Veterans Affairs Medical Center in Minneapolis Minnesota, has done countless research studies over many years.

One of Dr. Gannon's research studies in 2003 involved Type 2 diabetics (adult onset) patients who previously had not received any treatment for their diabetes. One group of patients consumed a regular balanced diet (15% protein, 55% carbohydrate, and 30% fat) and the second group consumed a higher protein diet (30% protein, 40% carbohydrate and 30% fat) for five weeks. The study revealed that the patients on the higher protein diet had a statistically significant improvement in both their daily blood sugars and the long-term measurement of their blood sugars.[17]

Translation: Increasing protein in the diet can improve your blood sugars for the short- and long term.

In addition to the above facts about protein intake, protein at meals and snacks enables the brain to communicate to your body that you have had enough food. Eating a piece of fruit between meals can satiate you for about an hour or two,

but if you add a piece of cheese or a few nuts, you will extend the satiety for another hour or two. The same holds true with meals. If you have a carbohydrate-based meal, it will hold you for maybe 2-3 hours, but if you add protein, it will keep you satiated longer.

Summary

Many people like to eat often, while others find it a nuisance to think about food every two hours. Personal diet balance is the key. So many health care professionals argue about high-carb, low-protein versus high-protein, low-carb diets. Both these types of diets do not seem balanced or effective in terms of health and well-being. Moderation in terms of eating adequate carbohydrate, protein and fat at each meal is the key, and the amounts needed differ from person to person.

Restoring balance to the body is essential for health and happiness. Protein is a key nutrient in the diet, assisting with making you feel full and happy, keeping your metabolism strong, and stabilizing your blood sugars.

From meats to nuts to dairy, there is ample variety in how you can take care of your body's protein needs. Check out the Recipes section for some delicious way to prepare and serve this major player in your health.

Fat:

The Third Major Player

Fat has been the most criticized food macronutrient of the last two decades. The message from many health care organizations has been the same: reduce or cut the fat.

The justification for this recommendation was a number of medical conditions, including heart disease, stroke, obesity, and cancer. The idea of fat as "bad" is uniformly endorsed by many Americans. They believe that the secret to a long and healthy life is simply to severely limit or cut fat from their diets. If only it was that simple! This chapter will give you the real skinny on fat.

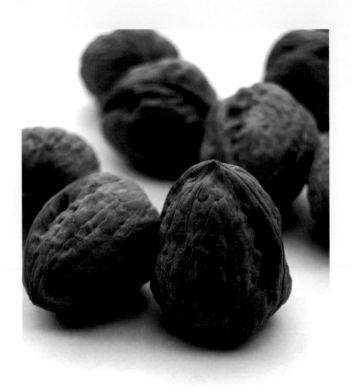

Walnuts: packed with monounsaturated and omega-3 fatty acids

The Great American Fat Frenzy

Walter Willett, M.D., of Harvard School of Public Health, stated it very well when he wrote:

> "The low-fat mantra has contributed to obesity. The nutrition community told people they had to worry only about counting fat grams. That encouraged the creation of thousands of low-fat products. I call it the 'Snackwell revolution.' Blithely consuming low-fat foods full of carbohydrates is a prescription for portliness, and any farmer knows if you pen up an animal and feed it grains, it will get fat. People are no different."[18]

Fact: Fat is an important macronutrient and has multiple functions in the body. It is so important that without fat, we would not be alive. Here are the reasons why:

- It supplies essential fatty acids the body cannot manufacture that are needed for healthy skin, hair and brain development in utero

- Fats are critical in the structure and function of all cells and the nervous system

- Fat is needed for proper digestion and absorption of fat-soluble vitamins (A, D, E and K)

- Sex hormones are derived from fat. Women who do not consume enough fat will have amenorrhea (lack of menstruation)

- Fat is a precursor to bile acids, corticosteroids (involved in the stress response, immune function, metabolism of food), and estrogen/testosterone, which are essential to life

- Sixty percent of the dry weight of the brain is fat, and healthy neurons contain a type of fat known as DHA

Fat provides nine calories per gram, making it the body's most *efficient* energy source. Fat digests in 4-5 hours and provides many essential nutrients. Yet despite all the good that fat can do for us, various health organizations recommend you restrict your fat intake to no more than between 20-35 percent of your daily calories. What exactly does this mean? For the last 25 years, the recommendation for fat, what type of fat, and how much fat to consume has dramatically changed, with most Americans not knowing what to do.

We have focused on fat recommendations and have forgotten what really matters: the balance of what we eat and how that affects us individually. Let's discuss various types of fats and then I'll show you how to apply this information to your food choices.

Just the Fats, Please!

The different types of fats are: **saturated, unsaturated, and trans fatty acids**. Fats are classified according to their chemical structure. Think in terms of a string of articles that are held together by chains. Fats are classified by the number of chains they contain.

The Chemistry of Fats

Saturated Fats   C-C-C-C-C
all links are full

Monounsaturated Fat   C-C=C-C-C
single double link in the chain (unfilled)

Polyunsaturated Fat   C-C=C-C=C
multiple double links in the chain (unfilled)

Saturated Fats

Saturated fats contain the maximum number of chains, which is where the name comes from. Saturated fat is found in chicken skin, fat around meat, whole milk, cream and butter.

Myth: Saturated fat is the evil villain to avoid.

Fact: If you look back at the research on fats over the last 80 years, limiting saturated fat or switching fat intake from saturated to other types of fats such as polyunsaturated has not lowered the risk of heart disease!

Findings from the landmark Framingham Study showed that after 40 years, those who ate the most saturated fat had lower cholesterol levels than those who consumed little cholesterol or saturated fat.

In 1992, Dr. William Castelli, M.D., director of the Framingham Study, stated:

> *"In Framingham, Massachusetts, the more saturated fat one ate, the more cholesterol one ate, the more calories one ate, the lower people's serum cholesterol...we found that the people who ate the most cholesterol, ate the most saturated fat, ate the most calories weighed the least and were the most physically active."* [19]

The U.S. Multiple Risk Factor Intervention Trial (MRFIT) studied the eating habits and mortality rates of 12,866 men.[20] The men consuming lower amounts of saturated fat and cholesterol only showed a marginal reduction in heart disease, but had a higher mortality rate. Clearly, something was amiss in shifting to a low-fat, low-cholesterol diet.

These studies are not a license for eating large amounts of saturated fat, such as fatty meats like prime rib. However, they do support the point of view that eating moderate amounts of cheese, butter and other foods containing saturated fat is not going to break your health bank and may add enjoyment to whatever you are consuming.

Unsaturated Fats

If the fat has fewer chains in the chemical structure it is known as unsaturated.

Generally, unsaturated fats are liquid at room temperature. If one chain is missing, the fat is called **monounsaturated** and if more than one chain is missing it is known as **polyunsaturated**. Foods containing high amounts of monounsaturated fat include olive oil, nuts and avocado. Foods containing high amounts of polyunsaturated fats include most vegetable oils such as corn, soybean, sunflower, safflower, and fish and fish oils.

Unsaturated fats can easily become damaged or oxidized when they are heated to high temperatures. Examples of oxidation include air turning a peeled apple brown or iron developing rust. Besides oxidation, these oils can become rancid when exposed to oxygen, moisture, or heat and therefore create more free radicals in the body.

Free radicals are byproducts or spin-offs of normal reactions that happen within the body and can be produced by pollution or tobacco smoke. Over time, an accumulation of free radicals in the body can contribute to heart disease, cancer, weight gain, immune disorders or premature aging. Therefore, it is essential when cooking with unsaturated fats that you only use them at low or medium temperatures.

One of the healthy oils that contains mostly saturated fat is **coconut oil**. An easy visual is to think of saturated fat as one that it is hard at room temperature. Saturated fats are the most stable to cook with, since they are not sensitive to becoming damaged when they are heated.

Besides being quite stable for cooking, coconut oil has other positive attributes: it contains a type of MCT (medium chain triglyceride) oil that is called *lauric acid*. The only other place you would find lauric acid is in mothers' breast milk. **Lauric acid is a powerful stimulant to the immune system, which may be helpful in preventing sickness.**

Free Radicals in the Body

normal/baseline
amount of free radicals in
the body

oxidation
amounts of free radicals with an
unhealthy lifestyle – smoke and
unhealthy foods

antioxidants
healthy foods decrease the
amount of free radicals in the
body

In addition, if you coat whatever you are cooking with olive oil prior to adding it to the pan, there will be less damage to the oil. If you are cooking at high temperatures, use saturated fats such as coconut oil or butter.

Monounsaturated Fats

Monounsaturated fats are healthy to include in your diet on a regular basis since they are associated with a lowered risk of heart disease. Monounsaturated fats can increase levels of HDL (the good cholesterol or H for happy), and lower triglycerides and LDL (the bad cholesterol or L for lousy) levels. When one's HDL levels are low, consuming monounsaturated fat on a daily basis can be very significant in increasing the level.

Avocados: packed with
healthy monounsaturated fats

When I worked at UCLA as the cardiac rehab dietitian, I would frequently see patients who ate a high-carbohydrate, low-fat diet and had low HDL levels and high triglycerides. Research had just begun to publish the connection between monounsaturated fat and HDL levels. I decided to test the research before giving recommendations to patients. At that time, my HDL was about 40-45 mg/dl, which is rather low for the level of my health *(see recommended levels in Diet, Disease and Medical Issues chapter)*.

Within six months of adding avocado and nuts to my diet daily, my HDL increased to 85. After that, I did another experiment. I refrained from eating nuts and avocado for six months, and my HDL levels lowered. Since that time, I eat adequate amounts of monounsaturated fat for my HDL to remain high. I started recommending this type of eating to patients who had low HDL levels, and I have seen multiple clients' HDL levels increase consistently by eating monounsaturated fat on a regular basis.

Healthy forms of monounsaturated fat such as avocados, nuts/seeds and nut butters can be very powerful in increasing HDL levels.

Polyunsaturated Fats and the Omegas

Polyunsaturated fats are another type of unsaturated fat. Two categories of polyunsaturated fats include omega-3 and omega-6 fatty acids. It is vitally important to differentiate between these two types of essential fatty acids, since they have entirely different consequences to your health.

There are three types of omega-3 fatty acids:

- alpha-linolenic acid (ALA)

- eicosapentaenoic acid (EPA)

- docosahexaenoic acid (DHA)

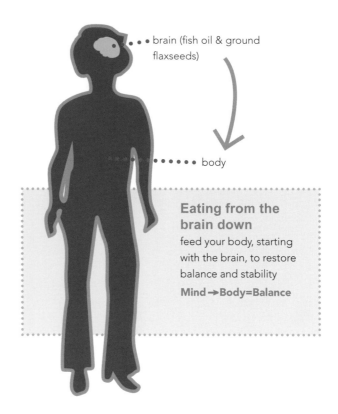

brain (fish oil & ground flaxseeds)

body

Eating from the brain down
feed your body, starting with the brain, to restore balance and stability
Mind → Body=Balance

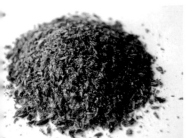

ALA is called an *essential* fatty acid because the body cannot manufacture it on its own, and therefore, one has to ingest the right foods to get it. The highest concentration of ALA is found in flaxseed, but it can also be found in green leafy vegetables and flaxseed oil. If you include one tablespoon of ground flaxseed in your diet per day, it will provide all your ALA needs for the day.

Ground flaxseeds: high in omega-3 fatty acids

Rich sources of EPA and DHA are fatty fish and fish oils. The American Heart Association recommends eating fatty fish at least twice a week to have a diet high in EPA and DHA. Salmon has approximately 300 mg. of DHA per ounce. Halibut contains approximately 80 mg. of DHA per ounce. Therefore, if you had a 3-ounce piece of either of these fish, you would be receiving 900 and 240 mg. respectively.

Consuming foods high in omega-3-fatty acids are associated with lowered rates of heart disease (including lowering of triglycerides, increased levels of HDL (the good cholesterol), lowered risk of inflammation in the body (which can decrease symptoms of rheumatoid arthritis), and lowered risk of certain types of cancers.

If you are not a fish eater, it is essential to take fish oil, either in oil or capsule form – since this fat *feeds* your brain. In order for your body to work efficiently, your brain needs to be properly fed or saturated with enough good fat. An average, well-nourished brain should have about 20 grams of DHA at all times, or about 20 fish oil capsules. If you consume the recommended amount of fish oil per day (see below), your brain will contain adequate DHA. Many health professionals now believe it is essential to feed the body from the brain down!

In prehistoric times, cavemen ate a Paleolithic diet consisting of large amounts of fish, and/or beef raised on grass (versus corn or grains) and therefore, ate larger amounts of DHA than the standard American diet, which provides barely 100 mg. of DHA per day.

Fish oil has become more user friendly in the last year. There's lemon-flavored fish oil, and other various flavors of fish oil that taste good. If you can't stomach the fish oil, many companies make fish oil capsules. Look at the back of the label for DHA and EPA content. The recommended amount is a minimum of 500-1000 mg. **each** of DHA and EPA. Many times the outside of the bottle states "1000 mg. of omega-3's," but does not give the breakdown for EPA and DHA. Therefore, it is necessary to read the back of the label for the exact amounts.

What to look for on a label:

EPA: 500-1000 mg.

DHA: 500-1000 mg.

You may have to take 3 or 4 capsules per day to achieve this amount of DHA or EPA unless the supplement you are taking has higher values or you are taking liquid fish oil which is more concentrated. If you take liquid fish oil, keep it refrigerated and use it within three months of opening.

Omega-3 fatty acids are essential since they have an **anti-inflammatory** effect in the body. It is now thought that because of the way animals are fed in the U.S., our diets have become deficient in omega-3's. If animals are fed grass, the products we eat will be rich in omega-3's. If they consume corn or grains they will produce omega-6 fatty acids.

Omega-6's

Omegas-6's are another classification of polyunsaturated fats, but they have a "**pro-inflammatory**" effect (increases inflammation) in the body. Research shows that 100 years ago, the ratio of omega-6 to omega-3 fatty acids in our diet was approximately 2-to-1.

Recent estimates show our food supply has changed the omega-6 to omega-3 ratio to 20-to-1.

This **large increase** in the ratio is what is believed to have caused a multitude of problems in our health. Having a higher omega-6 to omega-3 ratio is thought to have caused an increase in obesity, cancer, diabetes, and arthritis, just to name a few.

So, if you are consuming products from corn-fed animals (vs. grass fed like our cavemen) you will be receiving more omega-6 fatty acids. Since it is difficult at this time to find grass-fed meat – your best option may be to focus on ingesting your omega 3 fatty acids in other ways, such as increasing fish or fish oil supplements.

Oils rich in omega-6 fatty acids are: corn, vegetable, safflower, sunflower, and soybean. These oils are the ones we frequently see in processed foods because they are inexpensive. You cannot avoid these oils completely, but making a conscious effort to avoid processed foods and using olive oil on your salads and in your recipes will begin to shift the balance to higher levels of omega-3 fatty acids.

Going from Omega-6 to Omega-3

While attending a conference in Switzerland, I was surprised at the appearance of the cows there. Cows in Switzerland are pretty – a beautiful burgundy color, lean and frequently seen grazing on grass. This may sound strange, but after looking at overweight cows in America, the appearance of Swiss cows was surprising to me. In addition, the meat and dairy products tasted very different, and I found myself able to eat more than I regularly ate at home in America without gaining any weight. Since I was sitting at a conference, I knew this change had nothing to do with my activity level!

This observation sparked my interest in what animals are fed and how that **affects our health**. When animals are fed grass and allowed to graze out in pastures, they appear leaner, happier and produce products higher in omega-3 fatty acids. When fed corn or grains, animals produce products that are higher in omega-6 fatty acids.

Researchers state that our diets need to have more omega-3 rich foods than omega-6 foods. Shifting to a higher level or ratio of omega-3 rich foods is associated with:

- lower rates of heart disease

- lower blood pressure and risk of stroke

- improved immune function

- less risk of arthritis

- decreased incidence of age-related macular degeneration

- lower rates of dementia

Recent studies suggest that having an adequate intake of fish oil allows all the membranes in our cells to be more flexible. This flexibility improves blood flow, lowering risk of a cardiac event.

With respect to insulin resistance, fish oil has been shown to make insulin more efficient, which can lead to increased fat loss.

Having too high a ratio of omega-6 fatty acids in the diet creates the membranes of our cells to be stiffer and less permeable. Stiffness can lead to constriction of blood vessels, increased blood clotting, and an increase in sensitivity to pain. **When our cell membranes are inflexible, good nutrients cannot get in and waste products cannot get out.**

Studies coming out daily are continuing to show the benefits of fish oil and omega-3 rich foods. If you increase your intake of fatty fish (DHA, EPA) and ground flaxseed (ALA) for health, and decrease your intake of omega-6 foods, your brain and body will thank you!

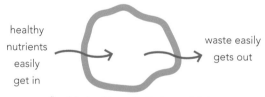

healthy nutrients easily get in — waste easily gets out

flexible healthy cells that are **rich** in omega-3 fatty acids

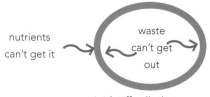

nutrients can't get it — waste can't get out

rigid stiff cells that are omega-3 **poor**

Omega-3 vs. Statin Drugs (cholesterol lowering drugs)

For those who are on statin drugs or considering this therapy, there is additional research of interest.

A 2008 study published in *The Lancet* looked at the difference between statin drugs versus supplements of omega-3 fatty acids on heart failure. After almost four years of follow-up, the group taking the omega-3 supplements reduced the risk of mortality by 9 percent and admission to the hospital for any cardiovascular cause by 8 percent. [21]

There were no differences seen in lowered risk of mortality or hospital admissions in the group on statin therapy. The research is becoming clear: important omega-3 fatty acids are lowering the risk of all types of inflammation. *(This is discussed in the Diet, Disease, and Medical Issues chapter.)*

Trans Fatty Acids: The Train of Destruction

Trans fat has received a lot of negative publicity lately. The FDA now requires food manufacturers to list trans fat on all labels. In 2006, New York City instituted a mandate for restaurants to avoid trans fat in their foods. Dr. Willett of Harvard School of Public Health calls trans fat from partially hydrogenated vegetable oil a "toxic substance not belonging in food." [22]

A trans fatty acid is an unsaturated fat that has a structure similar to saturated fats (with far worse health effects) through a process called hydrogenation. This chemical process is used by many food manufacturers to turn oils into shortening or stick margarine to increase the products' shelf life.

Trans fats are considered the most dangerous, since they can:

- raise LDL cholesterol
- lower HDL cholesterol
- raise triglyceride levels

It is now known that increasing one's intake of trans fatty acids can significantly increase one's risk for heart disease by as much as **37 percent**, well above any risk of consuming saturated fat.

A 2008 study published in the *American Journal of Epidemiology* found significant colorectal cancer in those with the highest intakes of trans fatty acids.[23] The study looked at 622 people who had colonoscopies at the University of North Carolina Hospitals in 2001 and 2002. Those ingesting 6.54 grams of trans fats on a daily basis were 86 percent more likely to have colon polyps than those whose intake was 3.63 grams or less.

To put this in perspective, a medium-size order of French fries has approximately 8 grams of trans fat, a small bag of potato chips has 5 grams, and a donut has about 5 grams. A regular-sized candy bar has 3 grams. If you eat even small amounts of processed foods, eating 6 or more grams of trans fat can easily add up.

Eating foods with trans fat occasionally may not pose a health risk, but think of how this type of eating can compound over a week, month or year – the damage done to your system could be insurmountable! Think of a food you like that is tasty and is contained in a package. How long can it stay looking and tasting good over a long period of time? This food most likely contains a fair amount of trans fat to increase its shelf life.

Types of foods containing man-made trans fat include cookies, cakes, crackers, chips, and other snack foods sold in markets or convenience stores that do not require refrigeration. If you cannot pronounce half of what is on the label, or the list of ingredients is too long to contemplate, think about how your body tries to process the "food." The following is a label on a cake from a grocery store chain that illustrates my point:

Filled White Cake with Buttercream Icing

Contains: sugar, enriched wheat flour (wheat flour, ferrous sulfate, niacin, thiamin mononitrate, riboflavin, folic acid), partially hydrogenated soybean and/or cottonseed and/or palm and/or palm kernel and/or coconut oils, water, milk, skim milk, corn syrup, strawberry apricot (sulfur dioxide), cocoa (alkali), contains 2 % or less of: salt, natural and artificial flavors, emulsifiers (propylene glycol monoesters, mono and di-glycerides, soy lecithin, sodium stearoyl lactylate, polyglycerol esters of fatty acids, glycerol mono-stearate, sorbitan tristearate, polysorbate 60), egg whites, corn sugar, modified foods starch, leavening (sodium bicarbonate, sodium aluminum phosphate, mono and dicalcium phosphate), cellulose, corn starch, high fructose corn syrup, carbohydrate gum, sodium citrate disodium phosphate, cheese culture, lactic acid, whey buttermilk, modified tapioca starch, sodium phosphate corn syrup solids, sodium caseinate, BHA, citric acid, potassium sorbate, sodium benzoate (preservatives), xanthan and locust bean gums, caramel color (sulfur dioxide), vanillin, beta carotene (color), FD &C color (reds #40 and #3, yellow #6 and #5, blue #1 and #2, titanium dioxide), vitamin D3.

Just imagine how hard your body has work to process this piece of cake with multiple ingredients. Not only does it contain many types of sugars, it also contains several sources of trans fat. I grew weary just typing the cake label, and I'm sure you did reading it!

Myth: When a label says "no trans fat" it is free of trans fat.

Fact: A manufacturer can make the serving size of the food so small, the amount of trans fat in the food is less than .5 gram per serving, which does not need to be reported.

However, if a person eats several foods per day with .5 grams each, that can easily add up to over 2 grams per day, which has been associated with an increase in heart disease. These fats are by far the most dangerous for the population in general, and especially for those at risk for heart disease or colon cancer.

Some foods such as beef and dairy products contain natural forms of trans fat that have been associated with possible health benefits. One such fat is called conjugated linoleic acid (CLA), which has been linked in helping decrease body fat, lowering inflammation in the body and increasing immunity. So far, the studies on CLA have been inconclusive, but we do know these fats are far different than man-made trans fats.

> The take away message: stay away from foods that have an extended shelf life, multiple complicated ingredients, and are overly processed.

Summary: Recapping the Fat Controversy

The subject of fat in food is highly controversial, with people on both sides of the extreme ends of the spectrum. The answer lies somewhere in the middle, and is individual for each person. In my opinion, if you balance your diet with good sources of protein and healthy sources of fats, the health benefits can be tremendous.

Consider the following:

- High-carbohydrate, low-fat diets have increased the incidence of obesity, and have not lowered incidence of heart disease

- High-carbohydrate, refined, low-fiber foods do not provide needed nutrients for the body and can increase incidence of insulin resistance in an already obese nation

By the same token, eating a high-fat diet without adequate fruits and vegetables does not provide enough nutrients to prevent many types of disease, including heart disease and cancer. Regular consumption of fat is part of a healthy balanced diet, including a large percentage of monounsaturated fat or omega-3 rich fats.

Over the last couple of decades, diets have changed, but it all comes back to informed balance. Don't fall victim to the "all fat is bad" frenzy. If you include healthy fats in your diet with some saturated fat and avoid trans fat, your supple arteries will thank you.

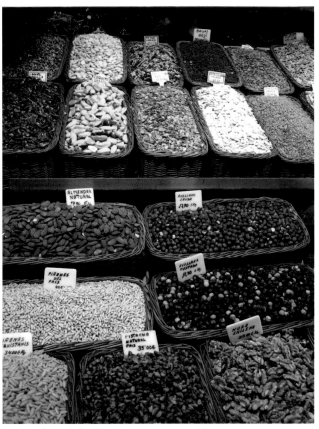

Nuts and seeds: high in monounsaturated fats

Beverages and Fluid Intake

We all know that most plants need regular watering to remain lush, green and beautiful. Once a plant is dried out, it is close to impossible to revive it overnight. If you add a lot of water to a dried out plant, it travels right through the soil. The dried out soil is like sand and does not easily retain water.

Your body works in the same way when it comes to fluid intake. Consistency is key: you can't go from drinking small amounts of water to consuming a large amount overnight. Many of us ration our fluid and then suddenly realize it is compromising our health. If you decide to increase your fluids and start drinking eight glasses a day, you may find yourself in the bathroom every hour on the hour! Increasing your fluid intake slowly is essential to restoring balance and health in the body.

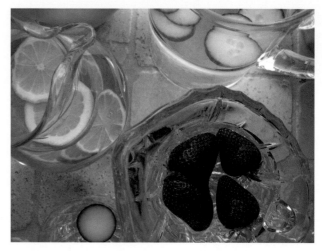

The Case for Fluids

You drink, therefore you are! Water is important because:

- It is the most abundant compound found in the human body as we are 60 percent water by weight

- All the important functions of our bodies depend on water since most nutrients are transported in water

- Our bloodstream is mostly water, as are our organs and tissues

- Toxins are released from our bodies in the form of urine and perspiration

- Water is a key player for proper digestion and absorption of nutrients

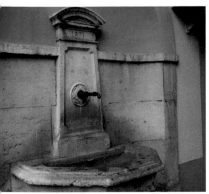
king fountain from 1871

The average male needs approximately 2,900 milliliters of water per day (12 8-oz cups) to maintain hydration. The average female needs approximately 2,200 milliliters per day (9 8-oz cups). Solid food can provide about 1,000 milliliters (4 cups) of water per day.[24]

Needs for fluids can dramatically change when considering different climates, varying levels of exercise, age, etc.

An easy way to determine whether you are receiving enough fluids is to check the color of your urine. If it is darkly colored, you are most likely dehydrated. Except for first thing in the morning, your urine throughout the day should be light yellow to clear. An exception to this rule is if you are taking vitamins, since vitamins can impact the color of your urine. Slowly increasing your fluid intake is important as it allows your bladder to accommodate more liquid.

"Feeling thirsty" is not a good way to determine whether you are properly hydrated, since **your body may already be two percent dehydrated by the time your thirst mechanism kicks in.**

Dehydration is dangerous since it can lead to headaches, dizziness, fatigue and a host of other symptoms. By the same token, it can also prevent health issues.

Jacqueline Chan, a researcher on the Adventist Health Study, found that men drinking five or more glasses of water a day could reduce their risk of a fatal heart attack by 50 percent.[25] This statistic is comparable with cessation of smoking. What a difference fluids can make!

The Explosion of Beverages: Think Before You Drink

Beverages are more popular than ever before, and we are a society that wants more and more interesting beverage choices. When I was a child, the common options were water, milk, coffee, tea and soft drinks. Today, there are countless choices with new beverages appearing every day. Many of these have added colorings, additives, sweeteners and non-nutritive artificial sweeteners, all of which can affect our health.

When I counsel my clients on beverages, they are disappointed at what I say: Stay with water, sparkling waters, or just plain water with slices of lemon, lime or cucumber since these are healthy fluids to drink.

It may seem boring at first, but water will save you calories, additional sugar intake, and increased sweet cravings resulting from artificial sugars.

In addition, sticking with water prevents you from ingesting large amounts of calories since the body does not register fluid calories as well as calories from solid foods.

Research conducted by Rick Mattes, Ph.D., R.D., on the cause of obesity in America showed that obesity is highly correlated with the increased intake of beverages. His research also indicated that solid food has a much greater affect on satiation than beverages. In his findings, Dr. Mattes wrote, "**Calories from solid foods are better 'registered' by the body than calories from liquids.**"[8]

When you think of how many beverages we have in our current food supply compared to 20 years ago, it is startling. Many people don't realize that the calories from beverages add up and do not have the same levels of satiation as solid food.

The following are examples of the calorie and carbohydrate content of some common beverages.

Beverage	Approximate Calories	Approximate Carbs
Mineral water/water	0	0
Hot tea with milk, 8 ounces	0-50	3-5 grams
Milk, 1 percent, 8-ounce cup	120	13 grams
Specialty water, 12 ounces	75	20 grams
Sports drink, 12 ounces	100-150	20-35 grams
Orange juice, 8-ounce cup	110	25-30 grams
Cranberry juice, 8-ounce cup	135	30-35 grams
Fruit punch, 8-ounce cup	120	32-35 grams
Regular soda, 12-ounce can	155	40 grams
Caffeinated energy drink, 12-ounce can	160	40 grams
Café latte, med-large	150-200	15-20 grams
Chai latte, med-large	200-300	40-50 grams
Mocha latte, med-large	250-550	40-50 grams
Smoothie drinks	500-800	60-100 grams

As you can see, many beverages contain a staggering amount of calories and additional carbohydrates or sugars. Even juices can contribute to a large amount of extra calories. Many clients lose weight by eliminating several glasses of juice per day. Remember, 15 grams of carbohydrate is equal to a slice of bread, so a morning coffee drink could be equal to three slices of bread!

Caffeine

About half of the fluid in coffee and tea can be counted toward your total intake of fluids. Coffee and tea do contain some benefits with respect to antioxidants. However, moderation of caffeinated beverages is important since consuming excess amounts can reverse the antioxidant benefits.

Excess caffeine can lead to high blood pressure, increased risk of heart disease, and insulin resistance. An 8-ounce cup of regular drip coffee has approximately 150 mg. of caffeine, while a cup of black tea contains approximately 40 mg. A cup of decaffeinated coffee has 2 mg. per 8-ounce cup. In addition to the antioxidants in tea, it contains an amino acid known as L-theanine that has been shown to counter the normal side effects of caffeine, such as high blood pressure and headaches. Therefore, tea may be a better choice than coffee for those desiring a hot beverage.

Alcohol

What about alcohol? Many studies have investigated the risks and benefits of alcohol. Harvard School of Public Health claims that alcohol is both a tonic and a poison, with the difference being mostly in the dose. Research has shown that moderate drinking can benefit those with heart disease. However, after closely looking at what was actually beneficial, it was discovered that resveratrol, a flavonoid (*see Phytochemical chapter*), found in the skins of grapes, was the phytochemical responsible for disease prevention. (*For more information on alcohol, please see the Diet, Disease, and Medical Issues chapter.*)

Calories do vary from drink to drink, but here are some averages:

Drink	Calories
Regular beer	140-300 per 12 ounces
Light beer	100-120 per 12 ounces
Single shot of liquor	110-120 per 1.5 ounces
Glass of wine	120-150 per 6 ounces
Mixed drinks	300-800 per drink

You can see how a few alcoholic beverages quickly add up, and in a moment of relaxation it's easy to lose count of your caloric intake. So, enjoy yourself, but be conscious of your choices. You can easily offset a week's hard work at a social gathering by drinking 2-3 glasses of wine, eating 3-4 hors d'oeuvres, along with the entrée and dessert.

Some tips for saving on alcohol calories include:

- Make your wine into a spritzer – half wine and half sparkling water

- Alternate alcoholic drinks with sparkling or mineral water

- If you plan on drinking, include alcohol in your daily allotment of calories

The body does not register calories from alcohol in the same way that it processes calories from food. Therefore, any calories consumed by drinking are additional to what you have already eaten that day. Since alcohol is digested as sugar, each drink can be correlated to having a slice of bread. Therefore, two glasses of wine is like adding two slices of bread to your meal.

Summary

It is essential to be conscious of how many calories your beverages are providing. You may find that you can take in as many calories drinking as you can chewing! Just as you would want to drive your vehicle with premium fuel, you want to put premium beverages in your body. If you have a favorite calorie-containing beverage, make sure to "exchange" it for something else you are eating so you don't overfill your tank.

If your body needs approximately 2,000 calories per day (an average for an adult) and you are including 300-500 calories per day of beverages, you are likely to gain weight unless you are compensating by eating fewer calories. One way to start educating yourself is to check labels for the serving size of the beverage (some contain two servings per small bottle) and then check the calories and carbohydrates. Lowering or eliminating calorie-containing beverages is one simple solution to managing your health and weight. And, remember to hydrate as often as you can with good old-fashioned water – just like your plants!

Sodium
What to Believe?

Small amounts of sodium are essential for proper health and functioning of the body. Salt (sodium chloride) is about 40 percent sodium by weight.

Salt has been around since the beginning of time and is used for many purposes, including flavoring and preserving food. Nowadays, our culture has become so used to the taste of salt that many people routinely add it to a dish before even tasting it.

Studies over the years show the importance of lowering salt for health, blood pressure, etc. The DASH diet is one study (see *Diet, Disease and Medical* chapter) that has demonstrated the health benefits of a low-sodium diet.

So, how much sodium can you have in your diet without compromising your health?

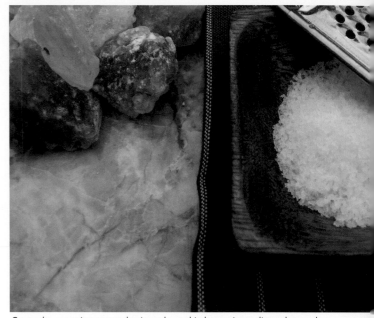

Sea salt: contains natural minerals and is lower in sodium than salt

The average adult gets about 6,000 mg. of sodium per day. Most health organizations recommend no more than 2,500 mg. per day. With such a discrepancy between these two numbers, is it necessary to limit your salt intake to this recommended level?

The answer is that for general health purposes, lowering your salt intake to no more than 3,000 mg. per day is prudent. If you have kidney, heart or other medical issues, it may be necessary to lower the level to 2,000-2,500 mg.

In order to lower the amount of sodium in your diet, you need to do the following:

Avoid or limit:

- **Processed and prepared foods** – we've discussed this in other chapters, but if you are eating a large percentage of foods from a box, can, or package, you're probably getting more sodium than you need. Choose fresh foods in their most organic form, such as fresh fruits, vegetables, eggs, meat, chicken, etc.

  If you are consuming something with a label, look at the sodium level. Stick to foods with less than 200-300 mg. per serving. If you lean toward fresh foods without a label, the natural sodium you receive from these foods will be minimal and adequate.

- **Condiments** – This includes adding table salt to your food (at 2,300 mg. per teaspoon) but also consider the amount in sauces, such as ketchup, barbeque, soy, or specialty sauces. Broths used in recipes can also add a fair amount of sodium, so I recommend you buy the low sodium types. MSG-containing foods have a lot of sodium in them, so it is best to avoid them.

- **Pickled, cured, smoked or preserved foods** – such as pickles, luncheon or cured meats

- **Fast foods** – just one fast food meal can add up to well over 2,000 mg. of sodium. If you eat at fast food restaurants, check the nutritional information available and choose options that are lower in sodium.

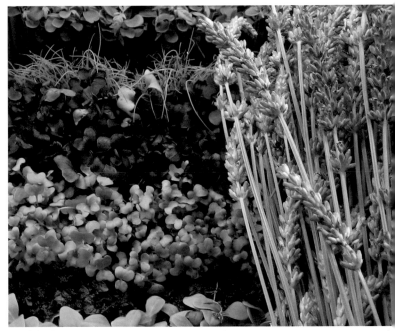

Fresh herbs: a great way to spice up your meals

Enjoy:

- Fresh or ground herbs as an alternative to salt

- Choose low-sodium alternatives (such as broth or low-sodium soup)

- Cut the amount of salt in recipes in half or cut it out completely

Sometimes it is unavoidable to have salt in restaurants and in social situations. Eating less salt may be hard at first, but you might be surprised how appealing the real taste of food can be. Part of restoring balance in the body is returning to whole, unprocessed foods. You'll be amazed at how much better you feel!

Balancing your Meals:
Putting it all Together

Now that we've talked about the three macronutrients – carbohydrate, protein, and fat – let's talk about how to combine them to work for your body and metabolism.

The way to combine carbohydrate, protein and fat to assist with weight management and health is different for each person. Curiously, many individuals neglect to look at the balance of their diets and focus mainly on vitamins to take or special foods to add. Simply making the effort to rebalance one's diet can solve many health-related issues from high cholesterol to acid reflux to insulin resistance.

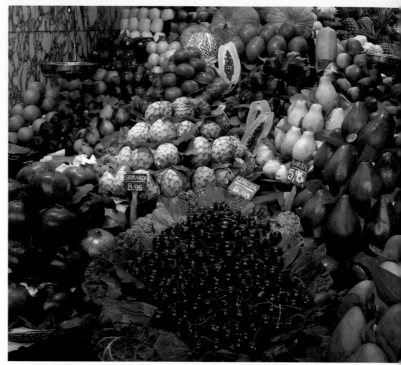

Mercat de Boqueria: Barcelona, Spain

A healthy way to put together a meal is:

- Start with a lean source of protein

- Balance it with a healthy source of carbohydrate, such as a fruit or vegetable

- Round out the meal with a small amount of monounsaturated or polyunsaturated omega-3 rich fat source

It's not surprising that nature knows best, and you'll find that many clean foods are combinations of the three macronutrients. For example, a glass of one percent milk contains protein, carbohydrate and a small amount of fat. Let's look at exactly what foods these macronutrient groups contain.

Carbohydrate

Carbohydrate containing foods are: fruits, vegetables, dairy products, nuts, seeds, whole grains, beans, and legumes. The amount of each food listed below represents approximately one serving of carbohydrate or 15 grams. As you may recall from the *Carbohydrate chapter*, 15 grams is approximately how much carbohydrate a slice of bread contains, as seen on a label. This list encompasses many foods that are classically counted as being a carbohydrate serving.

Healthy forms of carbohydrate (equal to about 15 grams of carbohydrate) – include these foods in your diet:

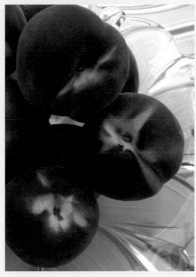

Peaches: contain vitamin C, potassium and fiber

½ cup of fresh fruit (citrus, melon, grapes, cherries, peaches, plums)

1 cup of berries (blueberries, strawberries, raspberries)

1 medium fruit (apple, orange, peach, etc.)

½ medium banana

½ large fruit such as grapefruit, papaya, large apple

2 cups of non-starchy vegetables (broccoli, cauliflower, zucchini)

10 cups of lettuce or mixed greens (romaine, butter, spinach)

½ cup of starchy vegetables (peas, beans, legumes)

½ cup of whole grains (brown rice and quinoa)

½ cup of beans (kidney, pinto, garbanzo, navy)

½ cup of yams or sweet potatoes

1 medium slice of whole wheat bread

½ cup of cooked steel-cut oats

1 cup of one percent milk

1 cup of plain yogurt

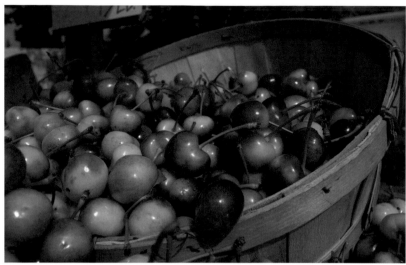
Cherries: contain flavonoids

Processed Forms of Carbohydrate (equal to about 15 grams of carbohydrate) – Limit these foods:	Other foods that contain approximately 15 grams of carbohydrate – Limit or avoid these foods:
1 medium slice of bread	½ cup of fruit juice (orange, apple, grape)
¼ of a bagel	2 small cookies
1 ounce of unsweetened cereal	1 small slice of unfrosted cake
1 corn or whole wheat tortilla (varies from brand to brand)	½ cup of regular ice cream
¾ cups of cooked cereal	⅓ cup nonfat frozen yogurt
½ cup of cooked pasta, white rice, potatoes	1 dollar-size pancake
3-4 small to medium sized crackers	1 tablespoon of maple syrup, honey, jelly/jam
1 cup of noodle or rice-based soup	Varying amounts of breakfast cereals, and desserts
1 crust of medium slice pizza	1 ounce of savory snack foods (potato chips, pretzels, etc.)

What about Spirits?

Alcohol is usually in a category all its own, but is counted as a unit equal to 6 ounces of wine, one 12-ounce beer, or 1.5 ounces of hard liquor. Since alcohol is digested as sugar, I count it as a carbohydrate unit, or 1 slice of bread.

Protein

1 serving of protein is 7-8 grams on a label. Normally we consume about 3-6 servings of protein per meal, or about 21-48 grams of protein. A unit of protein is equal to:

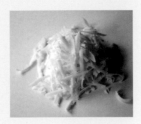

1 ounce of hard cheese (Cheddar, Swiss, Monterey Jack, Havarti, mozzarella or other hard cheeses)

¼ cup of low fat cottage cheese

¼ cup of part-skim ricotta cheese

2 tablespoons of parmesan cheese

1½ ounces of feta or goat cheese

1 cup of 1% milk

1 cup of plain yogurt

1 egg

2 egg whites

1 ounce of lean beef, lamb, pork, poultry, or fish

1½ ounces of shellfish (shrimp, crab, lobster)

¼ cup of canned tuna or salmon

¼ cup of natto (fermented soybeans)

¼ cup of tempeh

4 ounces of tofu or about ½ cup*

¼ cup of soybeans (edamame)*

2 tablespoons of raw nuts or seeds

2 tablespoons of natural peanut or other nut butters such as cashew or almond

½ cup of beans (kidney, pinto, garbanzo, navy)

* These soy products contain phytic acid (*see Clean Food chapter*)

Fat

One serving of fat is approximately equal to 5 grams of fat on a label. A reasonable amount of fat is 1-3 servings per meal. Approximately 5 grams of fat is equal to:

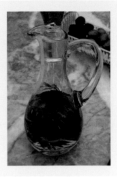

1 teaspoon of oil (olive preferred)

1 teaspoon of butter

1 tablespoon of salad dressing

1 tablespoon of cream cheese

1 tablespoon of sour cream

1 tablespoon of guacamole

⅓ of a medium avocado

Meal Ideas

Having a game plan for combining these food groups is important to health and satiety (feeling full). People are genetically programmed to have differing amounts of carbohydrate, protein, and fat so these are suggestions to get you started:

Breakfast:

- 2-4 servings of protein (or more if your exercise level is advanced or you have a larger frame)
- 2 servings of carbohydrate
- 1 serving of fat (if needed)

Breakfast Examples

Option 1:
- 2 scrambled eggs with ¼ cup of grated hard cheese and ¼ avocado
- 1 cup of fresh fruit or 1 medium piece of fruit

Option 2:
- ½ cup of cottage cheese mixed with ½ cup of ricotta cheese
- ½ cup of fresh fruit
- 2 tbsp. of raw or dry roasted nuts or seeds of your choice

Option 3:
- ¾ cup of plain low fat yogurt mixed with a ¼ cup of cottage cheese
- ½ cup of fresh fruit or frozen berries
- 2 tbsp. of raw or dry roasted nuts or seeds

Option 4:
- Frittata – medium square vegetable or meat based (see recipe)
- 1 cup of fresh fruit or 1 piece of medium fruit

Option 5:
- Smoothie: ½ cup of 1% milk, ½ cup of plain low fat yogurt, ½ cup of fruit or ½ medium banana, 2 tbsp. of protein powder (with no sweeteners and few additives), 1 tbsp. of natural peanut butter, crushed ice – mix in blender and enjoy

Weekend Option:
- 3-4 dollar size Ricotta Buckwheat Pancakes (see recipe)
- ½ cup of fresh fruit, applesauce, or Apple Blueberry Compote (see recipe)
- Additional protein if desired, i.e. 1 egg

Lunch/Dinner:

- 3-6 protein servings (or more if you are athletic or large framed)
- 2-3 servings of carbohydrate
- 2-3 servings of fat

Lunch/Dinner Examples

Option 1:
- 3-6 ounces of lean meat, chicken/turkey or fish (or other lean protein)
- Non-starchy vegetables and/or salad as desired
- ½-1 cup of whole grains and/or fresh fruit

Option 2:
- 3-6 ounces of lean hamburger or turkey/chicken burger without the bun
- Side salad with vegetables and avocado or a side of fruit
- Olive oil and vinegar on the side

Option 3:
- 1-1½ cups of chicken salad, tuna salad, or egg salad (see recipes)
- Piece of medium fresh fruit

Option 4:
- Mixed green salad with vegetables of choice, 3-6 ounces of lean protein, ½-1 ounce of cheese, ⅓ of a medium avocado, 1-2 tbsp. of nuts, and olive oil and vinegar for dressing (1-2 tbsp.)

Option 5:
- 1 square of high-protein lasagna (see recipe)
- Side salad or fruit

Option 6:
- 1 square of medium eggplant parmigiana (see recipe)
- Side salad with veggies

Option 7:
- 2 cups of chili (meat or vegetarian) (see recipes)
- Side salad or vegetables of choice

Snack:

- 1-2 servings of protein
- ½-1 serving of carbohydrate

Snack Examples

- 1 ounce of nuts (about 15-20) or seeds (varies) with a medium sized fruit
- 1-2 slices or ounces of cheese with medium fruit
- 1-2 tablespoons of natural nut butter and a piece of fruit or celery
- Hummus or guacamole (¼ cup) and cut up raw vegetables
- Healthy Nut Mix (¼ cup – see recipe)

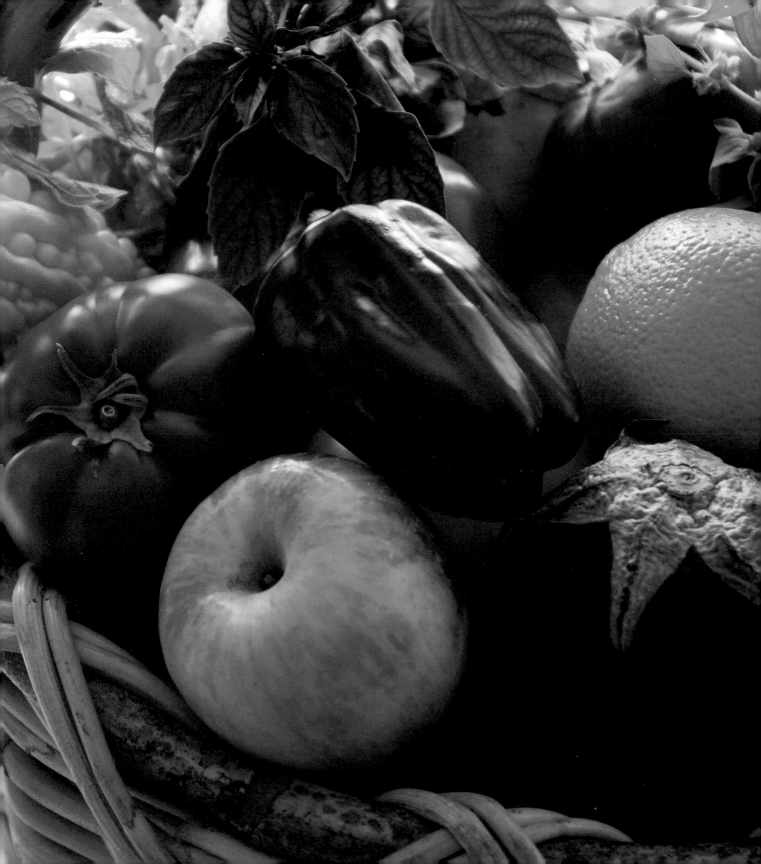

Part Two

Eating a *Clean*, Balanced Diet

Clean Food

For the very best diet, consider eating food that's "clean."

What does it mean to be eating clean food? Webster's Dictionary defines "clean" as free from dirt or pollution. In the nutrition world, clean eating is considered eating organic, unprocessed foods that are:

- pesticide-free

- hormone-free

- free-range

- grass-fed (versus corn fed)

- non-GMO (genetically modified organisms)

Eating clean is a process or a journey of slowly reducing the amount of manufactured processed food that you eat. Eating solely organic foods would be a difficult way to live in the world, considering most of us eat out or at friends' homes, but it is a worthwhile aspiration with a myriad of health benefits.

A good way to start eating clean is to avoid food in boxes or packages such as chips, crackers, cookies, donuts, etc. These contain refined, processed carbohydrates with trans fats or omega-6 fats, which do not have a favorable long-term effect on health.

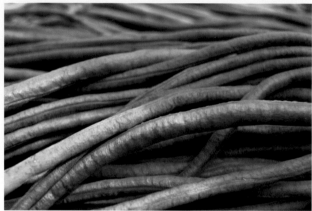
Green beans: good source of vitamins C and K

If you can afford to buy organic, free-range, or grass-fed food, these are the most optimal and can provide long-term benefits (*see Sorting Through the Grocery Store Maze chapter*). You might see a slight increase in your food budget now, but you could save on health costs later. Eating clean food is an investment in your future and in the environment.

Since a barrage of fake food abounds in America, switching your diet to clean, non-processed foods takes a conscious change. At first, this change can be quite challenging as you'll need to rethink your refueling process. You are starting a new way of shopping, cooking, eating and educating yourself. Reading labels takes time and effort. Don't get discouraged. In time, clean eating will become simple eating!

Clean Eating is a lifestyle choice. Once you choose this type of eating, you won't want to go back.

You Can't Fool Your Body

If you are wondering whether the extra effort and cost is worth it, consider this: processed foods can have an adverse effect on appetite, weight, and health. We've discussed how non-nutritive or fake sweeteners contain an unreasonable amount of sweetness to try to fake your body out. And, although your body knows it's not getting real sugar, it wants more sweetness, so these substitutes can actually trigger you to eat more sweet foods.

As we saw from the research described in the *Carbohdyrate chapter*, **most people who continue to use fake sweeteners will in time choose foods that are more and more sweet, rather than tasting the true flavor of food.**

Eventually, their altered taste buds become the filter that causes a false sense of perspective about food. I've had clients adding five or six packets of fake sweeteners to every food they were eating, and they still could not satisfy their endless sweet cravings. You don't want that to be you!

When reducing artificial sweeteners, you may find that it takes a few days of feeling intense sweet cravings and discomfort until your body settles down and becomes accustomed to less sweets. After a while, if you were to eat one of these foods, you would not like the fake sweet and chemical aftertaste. More than likely, you would wonder how you liked that food or beverage in the first place!

If a food label has more than five or six ingredients, you can usually put it in the processed food category (*see the cake label in the Fat chapter*), since it likely contains many additives or preservatives, additional sweeteners, and food dyes. Often, you can't pronounce most of the things you read on a label. Herein lies the clue! Foods with long lists of ingredients are probably not the healthiest to include in your eating plan.

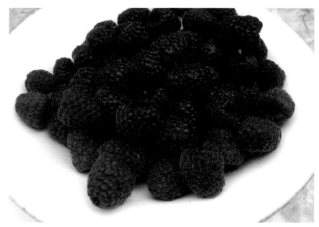

Raspberries: packed with vitamin C, manganese and flavonoids

When clients come for their initial visit, they may be trying their hardest to eat healthfully and avoid all the unhealthy foods they have been told are high in fat and calories. They may be putting "fat-free" half and half in their coffee or using "non-fat" nondairy creamer, not realizing that the half and half is full of sugar and corn syrup. The creamer has trans fat, although the label may mislead you, stating the food's "health" benefits.

Putting in a "real" food such as milk or even a little half and half is a far healthier alternative. **The little extra fat you are receiving is easier for your body to process than the manufactured processed ingredients.**

Balanced Eating Starts with Breakfast

Remember Jane from the *Protein* chapter? She skipped breakfast, only to be famished by mid-morning. Balanced breakfast choices are essential since they set the tone for the rest of the day. This is similar to how the shoes you choose to put on in the morning impact how your feet feel at the end of the day.

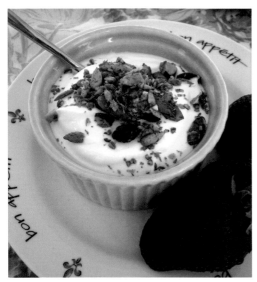

Plain yogurt topped with Healthy Nut Mix (See recipe)

Many health care professionals advocate breakfast cereals, including whole grain cereals of which there are a few. However, many breakfast cereals are full of sugar, additives and refined carbohydrates and are no better than eating a candy bar for breakfast!

Myth: Consuming a breakfast of whole grain cereal, milk and fruit is a very healthy breakfast that can carry you until lunch and sets a good tone for the day.

Fact: Consuming this type of breakfast contains a large amount of carbohydrate with very little protein and fat, which will not "hold" most individuals for more than a few hours.

Furthermore, the high insulin response to a large amount of carbohydrate can lower your blood sugar very quickly, which in turn increases hunger levels and the desire to eat more at the next meal. Eating a balanced breakfast with some protein, healthy forms of carbohydrate and some fat will balance out the insulin response and "hold" you for a longer period of time – usually until lunch, or 4-5 hours later.

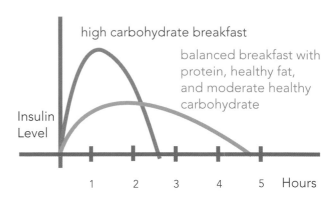

Let's look at how this fact played out with Bob.

Bob's Breakfast Blues

Bob was an avid exerciser and prided himself on healthy eating. He had started to gain weight around his middle and could not figure out what was happening to his body. He started his day at 8 a.m. with a large bowl of whole grain cereal, nonfat milk, fruit, a slice of whole wheat bread with apple butter and a small glass of orange juice. By 10:30 a.m. he was famished and had two pieces of fruit to hold him until lunch.

For lunch, he would have a turkey sandwich on whole wheat bread (hold the mayo) with a side of fruit. Dinner was usually a healthy, balanced meal with a lean protein choice, a vegetable, or salad or both and 2 cups of brown rice or whole wheat pasta. Most people would consider this regimen of eating balanced and healthy.

So, what was really going on with Bob, and how did we manage his blues? For starters, I suggested he check his breakfast against my food analysis program to see his exact nutritional intake. Here is the breakdown:

Bob's Old Breakfast (A):	Carbs (grams)	Protein (grams)
2 cups of whole grain cereal	82	11
1 cup of nonfat milk	12	8
1 medium banana	30	1
1 cup of mixed fresh berries	21	1
1 slice of whole wheat bread	15	2
1 tablespoon of apple butter	8	0
6 ounces of fresh squeezed orange juice	21	1
Total:	**189**	**24**

This breakfast was 853 calories with 83 percent of those calories coming from carbohydrate and only 5 grams of total fat.

Looking closer at the in-depth breakdown, **Breakfast A** contained:

- 83 percent carbohydrate
- 12 percent protein
- 5 percent fat

Bob was eating a whopping 12.5 slices worth of bread (189 divided by 15)! No wonder he was starving by mid-morning! When someone consumes this level of carbohydrate, their pancreas releases a large amount of insulin (the hormone that helps sugar to get into your cells), which causes your blood sugar to plummet within a 2-3 hour period.

Consuming that much carbohydrate in one sitting is the amount only an athlete who is exercising all day long could handle. Balancing your breakfast with healthy forms of carbohydrate, protein and fat is essential to starting off your day.

I suggested Bob reconsider his cereal breakfast and switch to 2 percent cottage cheese, mixed with some plain yogurt. I also suggested he keep the banana and berries and add some raw nuts and seeds.

Bob's New Breakfast (B):	Carbs (grams)	Protein (grams)
1 cup of 2% cottage cheese	7	31
½ cup of plain 2% yogurt	8	6
1 medium banana	30	1
1 cup of mixed berries	21	1
¼ cup of raw mixed nuts	3	3
Total:	**69**	**42**

This breakfast contains 550 calories, 13 grams of total fat, with 50 percent of the calories coming from carbohydrate.

Breakfast B contained:

- 50 percent carbohydrate
- 29 percent protein
- 21 percent fat

The revised breakfast contains 69 grams of total carbohydrate or 4.5 slices of bread, compared to 12.5 slices worth of bread. (There are approximately 20 slices of bread in a loaf.)

Now imagine how this plays out over time:

Slices of Bread:	Day	Week	Month	Year	Loaves
Breakfast A:	12.5	87.5	375	4563	228
Breakfast B:	4.5	31.5	135	1643	82
Difference:	**8**	**56**	**240**	**2920**	**146**

If Bob had continued to eat his regular breakfast for one year, he would have consumed 228 loaves worth of bread just at breakfast! No wonder he was gaining weight. By switching to Breakfast B he saved himself 146 loaves of bread and almost 44,000 total grams of carbohydrate per year. This just goes to show that **small changes in one meal can really add up and affect your weight and health!**

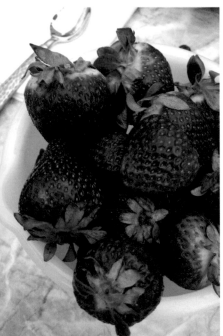

Strawberries: high in vitamin C and fiber

With respect to Bob's other meals, we added some healthy fats at lunch and altered his starch intake at dinner to 1 cup. He lost the extra weight he had gained, and he has continued to maintain his healthy lifestyle with balanced meals and exercise.

Although Bob had some changes to make to his diet, at least he was starting his day with breakfast. Many individuals do not take the time for breakfast at home. Instead they pick up a flavored, sugared coffee drink with a scone, not fully aware that they probably just consumed somewhere between 700-1,200 calories. Most of those calories are coming from sugar or refined carbohydrates, which sets them up for a very hungry day.

A few years ago, juice and smoothie places became all the rage. **People were unaware that a typical "healthy" smoothie contained anywhere from 500-800 calories with at least 90 grams of carbohydrate (6 slices worth of bread) in them.**

Even with limited time in the morning, consider how much easier and healthier it would be to eat a piece of fruit and a small bag of nuts or a few slices of cheese.

Beyond Breakfast – Clean Lunches and Dinners

For lunch and dinner, eating out has become the norm rather than the treat it once was (*see Eating away from Home and Weekend Eating chapter*). Better choices would be to choose items on the menu that are clean such as:

- grilled chicken breast, turkey, lean meat or fish

- salads with vegetables and protein added; olive oil and vinegar on the side

- a lean burger with a sliced avocado and tomato and a side of fruit or salad

- half a turkey/cheese sandwich with vegetable soup

- omelets with fruit/tomato slices or green salad

These choices are healthy and balanced, but can vary depending on the restaurant. Some restaurants are better than others and finding ones that don't add a lot of sauces and condiments (so you can add ones if you like that are healthier) are a better choice.

Ethnic restaurants are more challenging since they can add sauces and sweeteners. For example, Asian food usually has sauces that contain sugar and cornstarch. Therefore, **you may be receiving more carbohydrate than you realize in your "protein" dishes.**

Leaving Fast Food Behind

When you are starting a new way of eating, going to a fast food restaurant is not the safest thing to do. The temptations may be beyond what is reasonable for you. In the same manner, when you are learning a new way of eating, it may take some time for your taste buds to adjust.

Articles and books have been written about fast food and health risks. There are some healthy foods to be found at fast food restaurants, and most fast-food places are required to publish the nutritional information for their foods.

But, beware! Although fast-food restaurants have some healthy choices available, you may just default to your usual choices. In time, your fast food choices will become consistent with your new patterns of eating and will lead you to the road of health.

If you are traveling, it is easy to go to fast-food places since you are tired, the kids might be cranky and you feel like there is no other solution. With a little forethought and a cooler on hand you can pack:

- chicken, tuna, or egg salad in small containers (see recipes)

- hard-boiled eggs

- slices of hard cheese

- bags of nuts or seeds, or our Healthy Nut Mix (see recipes)

- cut-up veggies with hummus (see recipe) or guacamole

- containers of plain yogurt or cottage cheese

- whole fruit or cut-up fruit

Although fast food is a reality of our busy lives, eating meals at home allows you to keep your food clean and free of additives or preservatives, consistently maintaining balance in your body.

These simple lifestyle choices can add years to your life, given the healthier nutritional profile and added vitamins and minerals.

Little changes over time can create big differences.

Snacks

Have you ever noticed the strategic placement of vending machines? I've never seen one in a grocery store, library, or church. They are usually in schools, workplaces, or airports – places where you are stressed or have time to wander and eat. Vending machines are powerhouses for processed foods – chips, sugared nuts, donuts, granola bars, candy bars, etc. It is pretty close to impossible to have anything clean coming from a vending machine unless it is water or an occasional apple.

If you keep food with you at all times – little bags of nuts, a piece of fruit, or string cheese – you won't be lured by the machines. I always keep a bag of almonds in my purse so if I am delayed for some reason, the vending machines won't get the better of me. If I am traveling in the car or on an airplane, I'll pack fruit, cheese slices, nuts or some peanut butter with celery to tide me over to my destination.

Other So-called "Foods"

What about margarines? Margarines were developed in the early 1900s by researchers who hardened cheap oils into a food for the poor. Over the years, the look, taste, and appearance has improved considerably. Now, the food industry has us believing that margarine is actually heart-healthy. As Marion Nestle so elegantly writes in her book, *What to Eat*:

> *No matter what their labels say, all margarines are basically the same – mixtures of soybean oil and food additives. Everything else is theater and greasepaint.*[26]

Margarines contain trans fat. Even if the amount of trans fat is low, soybean oil is an omega-6 fatty acid or a pro-inflammatory fat and is not healthy except in small amounts in the diet.

Butter is a saturated fat and reasonable amounts of saturated fat have no ill effect on health. Enjoy a small amount of butter if you like the taste on food, and skip the man-made margarine. Most packaged foods contain some sort of margarine or soybean oil and therefore contain trans fat.

When foods have lots of additives, it can increase your craving for more food. For example, monosodium glutamate (MSG) is a flavor enhancer added to many foods. Most people think of MSG as something associated with Asian food. However, our food supply contains many sources of MSG that most of us are not aware of.

Hidden names for MSG or foods that can contain MSG on a food label are: gelatin, yeast extract, rice or brown rice syrup, malted barley, hydrolyzed vegetable protein (HVP), aspartame, hydrolyzed, glutamate, autolyzed yeast, and broth. [27]

Bottom line: Look at the labels on packages, containers and cans as you shop for groceries. The effort and time you invest in your own personal research will be time well spent, since you will be able to identify brands which are healthier.

Soy: Friend or Foe?

This brings us to the topic of soy. Soy was virtually unheard of until the early '90s except in infant formulas or for people with allergic reactions to cow's milk. Many food manufacturers joined the "soy bandwagon" since soy appeared to be the latest health food. I remember attending the Natural Foods Expo in Los Angeles and noticing practically every food manufacturer was promoting foods containing soy!

Years ago, I had to have a part of my thyroid removed. Soy nuts had become popular, and I started snacking on them. After a few weeks, I noticed I didn't feel so good. Since that was the only change I had made in my diet, I discontinued eating soy nuts. Within a few days I felt like my normal self again. At that time, I had no idea soy could interfere with thyroid function. A few years later, the research began to appear stating the negative effects of soy on thyroid.

Soy is not the health food many advocate. The studies regarding the health benefits of soy are very conflicting. Soy has been touted as a cure-all for hot flashes, heart disease, and cancer, just to name a few. Soy is also known as a "phytoestrogen," or a substance that mimics estrogen, which is significant, since estrogen can increase breast cancer in some women.

In 1999, two Food & Drug Administration (FDA) expert researchers on soy, Daniel Doerge and Daniel Sheehan, wrote an alarming letter to the FDA stating, "There is abundant evidence that some of the isoflavones found in soy, including genistein and equol – a metabolize of daidzen, demonstrate toxicity in estrogen-sensitive tissues and in the thyroid."[28]

Basically, they were stating that soy contains estrogen-like properties which can be harmful to many individuals and can also affect people with thyroid disease.

Despite this warning, the FDA approved soy as a "health" food and thus the soy craze began with manufacturers touting soy milk, soy bars, soy cereal, soy ice cream, and so forth.

In Asian cultures, soy is used as a condiment, rather than a "food." If you compare the American food culture to what Asians eat, you would have to compare many attributes rather than just one particular food. Asian cultures use small amounts of miso, tempeh and natto (about 2 teaspoons per day), which are traditional fermented soy products versus the unfermented soy "foods" Americans consume (about 1-3 cups per day).

Fermented soy foods have been used throughout Asia since 1134 BC. However, people did not eat unfermented soybeans. A number of health risks which have been largely hidden from the public, are now starting to surface regarding the safety of unfermented soy.

Unfermented soy contains high amounts of phytic acid, which blocks the absorption of minerals and nutrients in the gastrointestinal track. Among these are zinc, copper, iron, calcium and magnesium. With fermented soy, the phytic acid has been neutralized during the process of fermentation, which cancels out the negative properties.

Small amounts of phytic acid may not affect normal healthy individuals, but can affect children and older adults.

Unfermented soy can:

- Disrupt ovulation (thus interfering with getting pregnant)

- Promote breast cancer in some women

- Alter thyroid function or cause hypothyroidism (low thyroid)

- Lower sperm production in men

Soy protein isolate (SPI) is a far cry from the natural fermented soy, such as natto, tempeh, and miso. SPI is the powder that is in all the soy "foods" such as soy protein powder, soy milk, soy bars, etc. An interesting fact: many people think they are receiving calcium when they drink soy milk fortified with calcium. A few years back, it was discovered that the container soy milk was sold in absorbed most of the calcium, with very little left in the soy milk.

To make SPI powder, manufacturers take soybeans that are about 90 percent genetically modified, and mix them with a solution to remove the fiber. The soybeans minus the fiber are then dried at high temperatures to produce the SPI powder. [29] At this point, the protein in the powder is denatured -- or changed from its original form -- which means the original soy is no longer a good quality source of protein.

This powder is in most soy foods. If you like the taste of soy and want to include healthy forms of soy in your diet, you may wish to purchase traditional fermented soy foods such as miso, natto, or tempeh. Other forms of soy are associated with the health risks mentioned previously.

Say "No" to GMOs

The process of eating clean also requires being attentive to non-GMO (genetically modified organisms) foods.

What does it mean to eat non-GMO foods? The Center for Food Safety calls genetically modifying foods a "laboratory process of artificially inserting genes into the DNA of food crops or animals. GMOs can be engineered with genes from bacteria, viruses, insects, animals or even humans."

Recently I attended a lecture titled: *Is Our Food Safe: The Real Story About Genetically Engineered Food*. Jeffrey Smith, one of the world's leading experts on non-GMO eating, delivered a very informative but disturbing lecture on the health risks of GMO foods.

Why avoid GMO foods? Simply stated, changing the DNA of a food crop will ultimately change the way the food acts in our bodies. This could destroy the food's health properties and almost replace what is natural.

If a food product is labeled "certified organic" you can be assured there are no GMO products in it. Otherwise, it is necessary to check the labels for ingredients listed. What types of foods contain GMO components? The "Big Four" ingredients in processed foods are:

- Corn – corn flour, meal, starch, gluten and syrup, and sweeteners such as fructose, dextrose, and glucose

- Soy – soy flour, lecithin, protein, isolate, isoflavone, vegetable oil, and vegetable protein

- Canola – canola oil

- Sugar – anything not listed as 100% cane sugar

The complete guide to eating non-GMO food can be found at: responsibletechnology.org/GMFree/Home/index.cfm

This is a comprehensive shopping guide highlighting food manufacturers using only non-GMO products in addition to food products that contain GMO products.

High Fructose Corn Syrup

Media ads informing you that high fructose corn syrup (HFCS) is safe might lead you to believe that consuming a soft drink or food made with HFCS poses no health risks. When you look at the current research, however, nothing could be further from the truth.

To understand the truth, we need to look at the chemistry of different sugars and hormone interactions. HFCS was developed in the '70s from cornstarch made from genetically modified corn. This process results in a less expensive product than sugar, and is used by the major food companies to sweeten their products – anything from sodas to jams, ketchup, juices, and processed packaged foods.

Table sugar is composed of two sugars – glucose and fructose. All the cells of our body can readily metabolize glucose, but fructose is only metabolized via the liver. Large amounts of fructose going to the liver causes fatty liver, which leads to high cholesterol and triglycerides.

Since HFCS contains more fructose than sugar, the fructose is more readily available since it is not bound up with glucose, as is the case with natural sugar. Therefore, it has a straight shot to the liver.

When I was a child, candy was made from sugar. Now, almost every candy you buy is made from HFCS or corn syrup. If an individual is consuming foods containing HFCS on a daily basis, they could develop fatty liver over time. **Fatty liver increases the triglycerides in the blood, which in turn lowers the hormone leptin (remember leptin lowers your appetite). It is almost like the brain does not register the leptin levels, which causes you to continue eating.** If you want to consume something with sweetness, use "100 percent cane sugar" since it is non-GMO.

Other Tips for Clean Eating

One rule of thumb is to avoid food products with an abundance of preservatives and additives. If a food contains flavorings (including "natural" flavorings), emulsifiers, stabilizers, BHT, BHA, high fructose corn syrup, or genetically engineered or modified products, it is not a food that your body processes like a natural food or one that is in its simplest form.

Summary

It is challenging to go back to basics – eating clean and simple foods. Our food supply has dramatically changed. Apparently, manufacturers did not create enough profit by marketing food in its simplest form so they have changed the game – reaping more from consumers by adding sweeteners, additives and preservatives.

Eating clean and simple requires education, planning and organization to accommodate healthy balanced eating. Eating both clean and balanced is a process. You can start that process by reviewing all foods you eat, from snacks to meals, whether at home or at a restaurant. Break down and analyze each food.

Set small goals for yourself by first changing your breakfast since that is the most important meal of

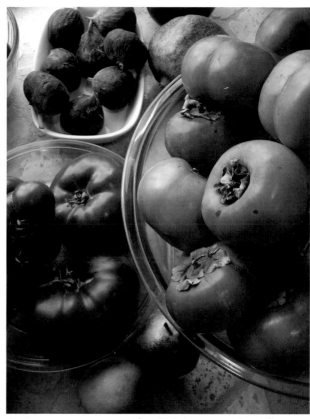

Persimmons, tomatoes and figs: high in vitamins C and fiber

the day. Then look at lunch and dinner including snacks, progressing to a week of meals.

When you are starting a new routine, give yourself time and room for progressing to healthy clean eating. If you try to do things too suddenly, the plan may backfire - kind of like going on a starvation diet only to end up binge eating later.

The *Organization* chapters will help get you started restoring balance to your life and body with easy tips for organizing your kitchen and shopping at the grocery store. Lifestyle changes take time, but commitment to the process will bring you the healthy results you desire.

Eating away from Home and Weekend Eating

People eat out more often today than they ever did in the past. In the '60s and '70s, the average family ate out 1-2 times per month, mostly for special occasions. That was my experience growing up. Now, with our fast-paced lives and increased food choices, it is typical for an individual or family to eat out 3-6 times per week.

For many of us, eating out is the norm, but it doesn't have to be a barrier to achieving your health goals. If you approach eating out with the same mindset you have in preparing your own meals, you can keep on track. Otherwise, one or two big meals out per week can sabotage your progress, even if you are highly disciplined for rest of the week.

Dining out can be a pleasurable and healthy experience if you know how and what to order. Two keys to success are choosing restaurants that offer a wide selection of meals and knowing what questions to ask.

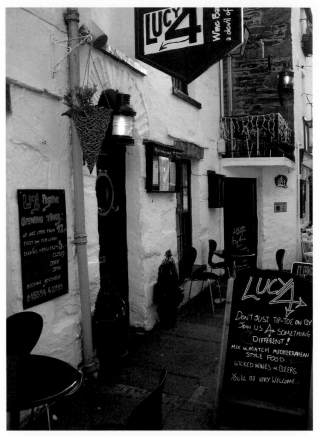

Restaurant in Lake District, England

Remember, you are the patron, and before you put any food in your mouth, you have the right to ask questions. Many people are afraid of being a nuisance, only to be disappointed when their food is served. Avoid the disappointment by being an informed consumer. It is more than okay to ask what goes into the preparation of the food because you care about your health and well-being.

Questions to ask your waiter or waitress:

- How is the food prepared – broiled, steamed, sautéed, fried, etc.?

- What comes with the main dish – vegetables, potatoes, French fries, etc.?

- What comes on the dish – sauces, dressings, or other?

- For Asian dishes – is there sugar, cornstarch, MSG, or other additives in the sauces?

Without a doubt, it is much harder to control what goes into the food since restaurants may use food additives, flavor enhancers, or additional salt and sugar. Asking questions can help you make a better meal choice. The wait staff may not be able to answer your questions, and you may need to speak to the chef. Often chefs like to come out of the kitchen and speak to patrons. If you are unable to get an answer, your best bet might be to order food or sauces on the side.

So where do we begin? The best place to start is to do pre-planning before you actually enter the restaurant. Avoid going to a restaurant when you are over-hungry. If it has been more than four hours since your last meal, eating a snack on the way to the restaurant is a good idea. Then, when the bread basket greets you at the table, you will be able to refuse or avoid the extra carbohydrates.

Tips to help with your dining experience:

- Having a small snack of protein like nuts or a piece of cheese an hour or so before is helpful in creating a level of self-control when ordering and eating

- Go on menupages.com, which is an online Web site offering the exact menu selections for many restaurants in most major cities. Also, many restaurants have their own Web sites with their menus posted

- Drink a glass of water when you sit down at the table just in case you are actually thirsty rather than just hungry

- Decide ahead of time what your body is hungry for and find something on the menu that matches. For example, are you hungry for foods hot or cold, hearty or light, crunchy or soft?

When you look at the menu, the wide range of food in some restaurants can be overwhelming. Knowing what you are actually hungry for and finding something that you want helps you make good choices.

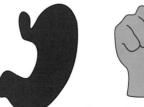

actual stomach and relationship to a fist

Your stomach is slightly larger than your fist.

In deciding how much food to order or consume, think of how much food it would take to fill the physical size of your fist. Ordering an appetizer, entrée, bread, dessert, and wine is most likely going to be more than your body physically requires unless you've run a marathon. Discontinuing your membership in the "clean plate club" is critical. Many of us were told that we needed to finish our plates due to the starving children in some foreign country. Eating only half of what we are served or eating all of it does not help any person in any country - especially ourselves.

It helps your humanity to eat half your entrée, package the other half and give it to a homeless person rather than eating the extra food.

Research confirms that people who eat with another person consume 25 percent more food than they would on their own, and 50 percent more food when they eat with a group of people. Peer pressure is an issue, even with adults. We want to appear part of the group and not deviate from what others are ordering, especially if the table is sharing food. Putting in your two cents worth may not be as hard as you think, and ordering a healthy entrée or appetizer for the table may be appreciated by others in your party.

Ease in Ordering and Eating

If too many things look good on the menu, try choosing one or two appetizers. Ordering a soup and an appetizer with protein in it, or ordering your own appetizer and sharing an entrée with a friend is usually enough for the average person.

Check in with yourself halfway through your meal to see if you are still hungry. If you're not sure, excuse yourself and go to the restroom. This will give you enough time to check in and assess your hunger levels.

Tasting your food is very helpful in knowing when you are satisfied and should stop. "Mouth feel" is a phrase we use in the dietitian world to have people really chew and taste their food. Research shows that if you taste your food, it will signal to your brain that you have had enough. When you eat your food without experiencing the taste, the signal to stop does not come as easily, which keeps you wanting more food.

Learning how to match your food intake to your metabolism is a skill that takes time and patience. Eating the 3-4 bites past satiation is just a habit. If you work at eating until you are no longer hungry, your body will get used to less. If you eat past satiation, your body will give you signals that it is not happy and you will feel uncomfortably full.

What Can Go Wrong?

Let's look at Tom. He was consistently exercising and trying to eat until satiation. When we looked at his food journals, he was eating about 200 less calories per day than he had been eating before his initial visit.

200 calories per day less x 7 days per week = 1,400 calories per week deficit plus the extra calories burned from exercising. Sounds good, right?

Well, on some weekends Tom would go all out and splurge, thinking it would be okay since he had been so disciplined during the week. Here is a typical meal he would eat on the weekend:

- 2 slices of bread with butter (250 calories)

- an appetizer of fried calamari (250-300 calories)

- an elegant entrée (600-1,000 calories)

- 2 glasses of wine (240 calories)

- dessert (300-700 calories)

You can easily see why all the work Tom accomplished during the week disappeared in one meal. His calorie intake was 1,650 to 2,500 calories, nullifying the calorie deficit for the week. When we figured out why Tom was not losing weight, we adjusted his weekend splurges so he felt he could still enjoy himself and lose weight.

Decide what the most important part of the meal is for you – what are you willing to forego versus what it is you need to be satisfied?

Tom decided he could not give up wine, and he needed a few bites of dessert. He could do without the bread and the calamari appetizer and order a more modest appetizer that included vegetables.

Tom's revised weekend meal:

- vegetable soup appetizer or a starter salad (200 calories)

- entrée with protein with vegetables (600 calories)

- 1 glass of wine (120 calories)

- a few bites of the dessert shared with friends (180 calories)

This dinner has about 1,100 calories. Tom decided to work out more on the days he ate more food, and eat a lighter lunch that day to accommodate the extra food the night he went out. After this change, he started to lose the weight he desired. He continues to enjoy eating out, but has limits as to what he orders since he wants to achieve his goal.

Weekend Eating

How about the innocent coffeehouse run on Saturday morning where you have your favorite grande coffee mocha drink with whipped cream and a large scone? This splurge could be as much as 1,000-1,200 calories, which is enough to stop you from attaining your weight loss goals.

A 2008 study at the University School of Medicine in St. Louis investigated how weekend eating can slow weight loss.[31] The researchers divided the participants into three groups and followed each for a year.

- One group lowered their daily calorie intake by 20 percent

- A second group increased daily physical activity by 20 percent

- A third group was the control group, which means they did not change their intake or exercise patterns

Before the study began, the researchers established baselines for an individual's eating and exercise habits.

They discovered:

- The calorie-restricted participants consumed the most calories on Saturdays, which hindered the weight loss process

- The exercise group ate more on both Saturday and Sunday and gained weight on the weekends

The researchers concluded that the typical weekend weight gain before the exercise or diet interventions would average nine pounds a year. This study demonstrated the importance of consistency in lifestyle changes. Unfortunately, even the most pristine eating during the week can be sabotaged by weekend eating.

Consistency across the board is important. We have all heard that changing your eating habits is more than a diet. It's a lifestyle. Eating fast food one day and a healthy diet the next confuses your body.

Summary

The bottom line is to stay on course with what you normally do at home. A colleague I work with once shared with me a wise expression: "Take your turf with you." If you normally eat protein at meals with vegetables or a salad, try to match that when you dine out. Consistent eating promotes balance in your body.

Judith Beck, Ph.D., whose father was the pioneer of cognitive behavioral therapy, has written several wonderful books on cognitive behavioral therapy and eating. In the seminars she leads for health care professionals, she speaks about thinking of your life changes in terms of a "full dose." [32] For example, if a doctor tells you to take an aspirin a day, you wouldn't take a quarter of that dose. You would take the full amount. If you have a bacterial infection, you take the full course of antibiotics so the medication can be effective.

In the same light, giving your body the "full dose" of lifestyle eating requires taking the plan of what you have decided is healthy for you, and staying with it, even when you dine out and during special occasions.

Part Three

Weight Management

Listening to your Body
Developing Hunger Awareness for Life

Hunger and satiation have been the subject of many studies in the last 10 years. At their core, these are very complex issues – physically, hormonally and biochemically. Presently, researchers are attempting to identify what physical attributes are responsible for levels of hunger and the desire to eat.

Current culture and oversized restaurant portions mean the average American is eating larger servings of food than he or she would have 30 years ago. In his 2006 book, *Mindless Eating: Why We Eat More Than We Think*, Brian Wansink of Cornell University's Food and Brand Lab details how making more than 200 food decisions a day can switch us into automatic pilot where we operate in a "mindless" mode of eating large portions and comfort food. [33]

In the 2004 documentary film "Supersize Me," Morgan Spurlock demonstrated what happens when a man of normal weight consumes only McDonald's meals for 30 days. It was amazing to watch and at the same time sobering to see the decline in his vitality and energy. Just as disturbing were his dangerously high levels of cholesterol, triglycerides, and blood sugars during the 30 days of eating a limited diet of only fast food. After this film debuted, McDonald's eliminated their

supersize portions. However, Americans continue to eat much larger portions than any other nation and is the country with the highest obesity rates in the world!

Portion sizes in homes and restaurants in many other countries are smaller than the U.S. Furthermore, people tend to eat larger breakfasts, which helps with satiety later in the day.

The Hunger Hormones: Insulin, Ghrelin and Leptin

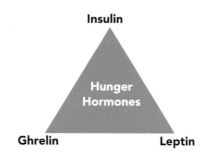

Our hormones affect our hunger. Insulin resistance *(see Carbohydrate chapter)*, is a syndrome where the insulin does not respond normally, allowing blood sugars (glucose) to enter the cells. It is almost as if the hormone insulin is sleepy or sluggish (hence the term resistant). Since the insulin is not allowing the glucose to easily enter the cells, you can experience hunger or the desire to eat, even though you are not physically hungry.

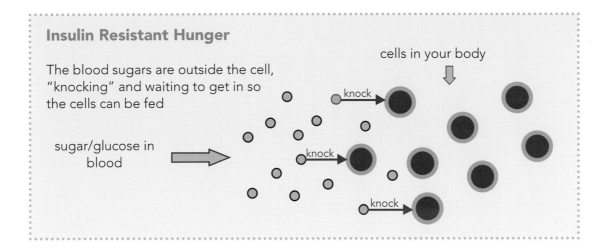

Insulin Resistant Hunger

The blood sugars are outside the cell, "knocking" and waiting to get in so the cells can be fed

cells in your body

sugar/glucose in blood

knock

knock

knock

For example, if you consume high carbohydrate meals on a regular basis that are not balanced with respect to protein and good fat, you may continually crave carbohydrates. You begin with one piece of bread at the restaurant and soon you have consumed three slices of bread before your meal arrives. Or you eat a few chips at a party, only to find yourself eating a good portion of the bowl. Even though you are not physically hungry, your body gives you the signal to eat even though you've had enough food.

Often you know what you are "supposed" to be eating, but the body continues to give you the signal to eat more carbohydrates. This signal keeps perpetuating. The more carbohydrates you consume, the more your energy levels fluctuate between high and low throughout the day. Consequently, you never truly feel like you are running on real energy.

When an insulin resistant person consumes a high-sugar or high-carbohydrate diet, there is an abundance of sugar or glucose in their system. When glucose waits outside the cells, knocking and waiting to get in, it creates a desire to eat many times during the day. If you are aware of this and realizes it is not true hunger and only a physical

desire to eat due to your biochemistry being out of balance, you can change the system. If you wait long enough, usually within an hour, your desire to eat simply can disappear. To calm the system down, and feel true hunger and satiation, requires diligence. Food cravings increase, but eventually will subside.

In addition, your body prefers carbohydrates or glucose as its primary fuel. Therefore, if you are eating a very high carbohydrate diet, your body will first turn to utilize the carbohydrate before tapping into calories from fat or protein. To make matters worse, you may not tap into utilizing your fat stores if you are on a plan to lose weight. If you continue to eat a high-carbohydrate or high-sugar diet, your body will prompt you to continue eating these foods, leading to chronic carbohydrate cravings. When blood sugars stay elevated, your body continues to secrete insulin, the hormone that unlocks the cell for sugar to get in. Insulin is also the hormone that stores fat. Therefore, if the insulin levels stay elevated, your system can store the extra carbohydrate as fat, rather than being used as fuel for energy.

Leptin and Ghrelin

As discussed in the *Protein chapter*, the hormones leptin and ghrelin also affect appetite and the desire to eat. Leptin turns off the hunger mechanism and ghrelin turns it on (remember leptin *lowers* the appetite and ghrelin *grows* it). The balance of how we eat the macronutrients of carbohydrate, protein and fat influences the levels of leptin and ghrelin. Learning how your individual body functions and how much protein you need to lower your ghrelin to lessen your appetite is worth exploring.

Knowing how these hunger hormones work can help reset hunger levels back to baseline levels, perhaps even close to levels during infancy.

The Hunger Scale: Resetting your Stomach

One useful tool to utilize is the Hunger Scale, which has a 10-point rating system. Zero means a person is ravenous, over hungry, or simply empty. This is the "point of no return." A person at this point literally wants to cram as much food in his or her mouth as quickly as possible. Unfortunately, when our bodies become this hungry, the blood sugar has dropped, resulting in overeating past the point of satiation into fullness or stomach pressure. In this case, the individual having the cravings does

not "feel" better or satisfied until he or she has eaten well past physiological satiation.

The upper end of the scale is 10 or "Thanksgiving full" or "food coma." The middle of the scale, 5-6, is physiologically satisfied or comfortable, neutral or "just right." At the low end, 3-4 is slightly hungry and 1-2 means physiologically hungry and ready to eat. As we move up the scale, 6-7 is full and 8-9 is stomach pressure.

Research shows that the average overweight person may eat only about 50-100 more calories per day than they physically need. This might register as a 6-½ or 7 on the Hunger Scale. Many times we think we are eating "so much," or see those who that are very overweight and think they eat abundantly, when in reality they may be eating only a few bites more per meal or per day than their metabolism requires.

If we reverse this process and honor our hunger and satiation signals, leaving a few bites on our plates, we may lose the weight gained over a period of time. However, many make an instant decision that the weight "must come off right now," and find the nearest, most convenient diet center or program. These diets typically provide meals or instructions for low calorie diets (normally less than 1,200 calories per day) which can drop a person into a semi-starvation or starvation mode.

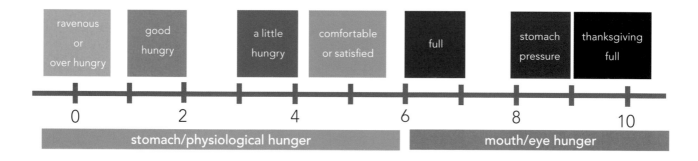

The Extra Bites Add Up

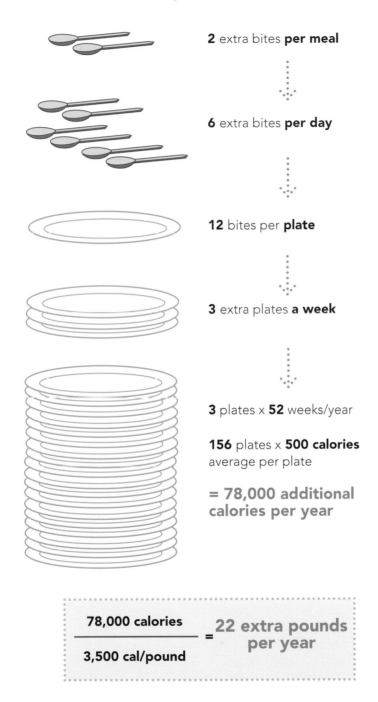

2 extra bites **per meal**

6 extra bites **per day**

12 bites per **plate**

3 extra plates **a week**

3 plates x **52** weeks/year

156 plates x **500 calories** average per plate

= 78,000 additional calories per year

$$\frac{78{,}000 \text{ calories}}{3{,}500 \text{ cal/pound}} = \textbf{22 extra pounds per year}$$

Take a look at how consuming a few extra bites over a year can add up. The numbers may look pretty daunting at first, but when you look at the opportunity it presents, this is actually good news! Eating two teaspoons **less** per meal creates a huge impact on lowering your weight – what do you have to lose?

The stomach has what athletes term "muscle memory." If you walk a certain way, you will walk that way unless someone asks, "Why do you walk that way?"

We become accustomed to eating a certain amount of food via the muscle memory of the stomach and will default to that amount unless we retrain or re-set the stomach to get used to less food. This skill requires attentiveness and **can** be done over a period of time. Many health care professional have called this "eating mindfully."

To use the scale to reset the muscle memory of the stomach, a person might start eating at 1-2 and then check in with themselves at 3-4 by asking, "How many more bites will it take me to get to 5-6? Two more bites, three more bites, or just one?" When someone reaches the point when they are no longer hungry, this is the point to stop – this may feel nebulous or uncomfortable at first.

Sometimes it is wiser to stop eating when you are not sure if you are hungry or full and trust you are satisfied. If you do this long enough (at least 20 meals in a row), your body will begin to give clear signals of hunger and satiation.

It may feel like your body is actually fighting with you since you have consumed more food in the past. As your fork pierces one more bite, this is the time to distract yourself by leaving the kitchen or dining area, or engaging in something you like to do as your default response to eating changes. Over time, you will retrain your stomach to eat less food. The smaller amount of food will satisfy the muscle memory of the stomach. After this adjustment takes place, eating more will cause you to feel very uncomfortable.

Many health care professionals identify eating from 0-6 physiological or "stomach hunger," and eating from 6-10 as "mouth or eye hunger." Mouth hunger is only a sensation in the mouth to eat or a craving. Many people think they need to respond to cravings. However, just being aware that wanting to eat is a craving and it is not necessary to respond to this feeling, can start changing the signals your body gives you in terms of wanting to eat more food. With diligence, eating less will become a new default resulting in the body returning to a normal weight.

Helpful hints on this journey:

- Make sure you are hydrated since sometimes you may perceive you are hungry when you are actually thirsty and/or dehydrated

- Take the time to eat in a calm environment, sitting down, even if it is for 10-15 minutes to allow for proper digestion and absorption

- Slowly chew and savor each bite since the extra taste in your mouth will signal to your brain that you have had enough to eat

- Recognize no easy solution exists. Take time to find the right balance, which ultimately leads to achieving success

Marcie's Story: Lesson Learned

Marcie's story illustrates how she learned to balance her eating and hunger awareness. She came in for a nutrition consult following her freshman year in college after gaining more than the "Freshman 15." (This is the nickname given to the phenomenon of putting on weight during the first year of college.)

In high school, I could eat anything and stay stick thin. Despite the challenges of my three family members to keep their weights down, I remained the thin one. I ate bread, fried foods, and desserts. I ate everything fattening. Nothing made a difference - until I entered college.

My freshman year in Philadelphia, I continued to eat whatever was in front of my face. My diet of cafeteria food, easy mac and beer did not sustain my figure like it did in high school. By the end of my freshman year I had gained 20 pounds. Translate that into a 5'2" frame and you get pants that don't fit and nights of crying to your mother, "I am now officially fat!" She empathized and sent me to Susan.

When I walked into Susan's office, I didn't realize exactly how much weight I had gained. Luckily, Susan did not stress weight as an issue. What she did stress was how she was going to help me, not with a diet, but with a lifestyle. We started with what foods I liked and didn't like, and what were better choices. I understood the effects each glass of beer, hamburger or iced mocha had on my small frame and what my mind was telling me versus what my body needed.

Over the course of the summer I saw Susan weekly, and we worked together on my mind and body. I could eat the foods I liked, but I had to get in touch with why I was eating and that I didn't need to eat until I was full. "Stop eating when you are comfortable," Susan said. As simple as this sounds, it's extremely difficult to know what feels comfortable. For me, there's a very slim line between hungry and not hungry.

As I learned to identify the reasons for my hunger and how to control it, I gradually reduced my carbohydrate intake and beer drinking. I increased my workouts. I stopped eating when I was comfortable. Finally I could leave food on my plate! It was a challenge. We also explored reasons for eating such as stress and loneliness. By the end of the summer, I was even more aware and weighed 15 pounds less.

Leaving Susan to go back to college was extremely difficult. I was fearful. Could I really do this on my own? I was going back to frat parties, late nights, the student budget, the less health-conscious East Coast. Susan assured me that I would be fine because I had the tools and determination. I inhaled Susan's confidence and inspiration and went east. I reduced my alcohol consumption. I forced the workouts to fit my class schedule. I stopped eating bread with my sandwiches and hamburgers. I maintained, and then lost about five more pounds.

Now, four years later I am living in New York City. I face new challenges. Every corner has a pizza place, a donut shop, or bagel emporium. The city is one huge living breathing carb! I eat a bagel on Saturday mornings, but then I make sure I walk 5-10 miles around the city. I indulge on wine and cheese, but watch myself more carefully throughout the week. I remember the importance of my lifestyle changes. I pay attention to why I'm eating and what I'm eating. I know I can live in NYC and never let myself blow up again. Sometimes I catch a reflection of myself in a store front window and smile, remembering that sorry summer that will never resurface again.

Marcie learned how to balance her food, hunger levels, and the importance of exercise. The lifestyle changes she learned in her youth will carry her throughout life.

Summary: Hunger is one of the main keys to weight management

Besides getting a proper balance in the diet, eating from hunger until satiation is one of the primary keys for weight and medical management. We've addressed balance in the diet, and future chapters will address exercise, sleep, stress, lifestyle changes, medical issues and the effect of medications.

Dieting, Skipping Meals and Starvation

It's a plain and simple fact that quick and permanent weight loss is non-existent. Weight management is good, old-fashioned hard work. Sometimes the weight comes off easily, but more often than not, intense focus and dedication are required to reach the goal.

The key to achieving weight goals is a lifestyle journey. If I were to say this any differently, it would be misleading. It's a journey accessible to everyone and is worth taking for its long-term rewards. For many, a combination of receiving help from competent health care professionals and being open and ready to change will facilitate the process.

Weight is more than just calories in and calories out. For health gurus to reduce such a complex process to an equation is not realistic for those struggling with their weight.

Often people hear messages such as:

- "Just watch your diet"
- "Just push away from the table"
- "Just be more active"
- "Just eat less and exercise more"

So many "justs!" If losing weight was as simple as any of these well-meaning, but not practical suggestions, there would not be a weight epidemic in America, where approximately one in three adults is overweight.

The dieting process has a 95 percent failure rate, yet many still hold out for that "one last time." Noted registered dietitian Dana Armstrong put it this way: "How would you feel if you failed at something over and over again and the experts kept prescribing a treatment with a 95 percent failure rate, then blamed you when it didn't work?"

Dieting does not work – lifestyle change does and this concept needs to be conveyed to the public at large.

So, where do we begin helping those who need or want to lose weight? One of the first things is to address hunger and satiation (*see Hunger chapter*).

Part of the non-dieting approach I advocate is learning how to recognize signs of physiological hunger so that you begin a meal when you are truly hungry, and end it when you are actually satisfied.

The behavior of eating from true physiological hunger can be one of the most difficult components to learn because there are so many factors affecting hunger/eating/satiation/fullness. Emotions, balanced meals, activity level, brain chemistry, behavioral patterns, and eating disorders all affect this process.

Dieting and Missing Meals

Most diet programs rely on low-calorie foods and/or low-calorie meals that are typically less than 1,200 calories per day. Our metabolisms and nutrient needs cannot be satisfied with this meager amount of calories on a regular basis. When we fall below 1,200 calories per day our bodies try to compensate and adjust by dropping our metabolic rate, typically slipping into "starvation mode."

This starvation mode lowers metabolism and throws the body into a yo-yo pattern commonly seen with diets. *Giving our bodies dignity* to change slowly helps with long-term success. It may be a matter of eating fewer bites at each meal and slowly increasing the activity level so the metabolism is not compromised and fat loss (rather than fat and muscle loss) can occur.

Some have experienced multiple diet failures before giving up and saying, "This isn't working" and then moving into a mindset of acceptance that there is no quick fix. With that understanding, the real journey of maintaining a healthy lifestyle and weight loss can now begin. The key is not succumbing to the failure, but rather seeking out success through understanding your own body, with some help from a trained professional.

What happens when you chronically skip meals? After eating a meal, metabolism increases. In the scientific community this is called *thermogenesis*, or the thermic effect of food. Beverages or food are placed in thermoses to keep them hot until we are able to consume what is contained in them. This concept is true for food. Eating increases metabolism, or heat produced in your body, to digest or break down the food.

If you skip a meal, your metabolism will drop down below baseline and will not increase again until you eat your next meal. Just think what happens if you don't eat breakfast or lunch and wait until dinner. Your metabolism is basically in the drain for the entire day; it increases at night; and then drops later in the night when you sleep. With this regimen, your metabolism only elevates between dinner and bedtime, or for 4-6 hours a day. It is easy to see how weight can quickly increase with this regimen.

Regular meals spaced throughout the day are essential to maintaining a healthy metabolism and natural weight.

Increased metabolism = thermogenesis

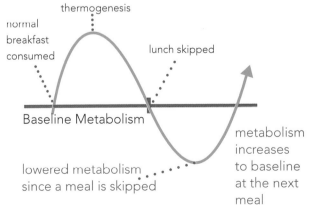

normal breakfast consumed

thermogenesis

lunch skipped

Baseline Metabolism

lowered metabolism since a meal is skipped

metabolism increases to baseline at the next meal

The Seriousness of Starvation

A starvation study, known as the Keys study, was done in 1944-1945. Five years later, Ancel Keys wrote *The Biology of Human Starvation*, which described the physical and personality changes of 32 men who took part in the Minnesota Experiment of starvation rather than go to war. [34]

This group of wartime conscientious objectors agreed to a semi-starvation diet that averaged 1,570 calories per day compared to more than double the calorie level during the control period or normal eating period. The men were required to lose an average of 24 percent of their body weight by food restriction. They were also required to sustain vigorous physical activity (walking approximately 22 miles per week), in addition to walking to and from the dining hall, which added another two to three miles each day.

Physical changes in the men included:

- Lowered metabolism by close to 40 percent by the end of the six month period

- Abnormal accumulation of fluid around the ankles and wrists called edema, which is linked to starvation

- Decreased work capacity, including limited ability to walk long distances or stand for long periods

- Lower tolerance for cold (all the men frequently complained of cold hands and feet, even in mid-July after wearing jackets all day and piling on blankets at night)

- Hair changes in which the hair became thin, dry, or lost

Psychological/personality changes that occurred included:

- An increased incidence of apathy, depression, and tiredness

- A marked decrease in self-discipline, mental alertness, comprehension, and ambition

- A decrease in sexual interest and loss of libido

- Personal appearance and grooming deterioration

- A high level of nervousness, restlessness and anxiety

Keys also noted a marked increase in food preoccupation. Many of the men spent time collecting recipes, studying cookbooks, and planning about how they would spend the day's food allotment. The men became possessive about their food, eating to the last crumb and licking their plates. They demonstrated extensive gum chewing, increased coffee/tea consumption and nail biting.

There was deterioration in social activities within the group with the tone becoming sober, serious and sarcastic. The men were hyper-irritable. During the re-feeding (increased calories) period, hunger pangs were reported as more intense than ever. The men's appetites were insatiable, and they reported wanting more food, even when they were physically full. The men continued to lick their plates, with most of them not eating normal amounts of food until Week 33 of re-feeding. In terms of physical changes, the men gained fat tissue rapidly with lean tissue recovering more slowly. The men had problems with constipation, stomach pains, heartburn and gas, especially when they overate.

This study is not widely circulated among the

medical community, but should be taken seriously as the findings are relevant to how people diet today. Since the '70s, many people have undertaken extreme diets and wonder why they have trouble with depression, bingeing, and preoccupation with food, in addition to large decreases in metabolism. This mid-century study illustrates the detrimental short and long-term effects of dieting. You can stop the bleeding, but that does not necessarily mean you will not see a scar later.

The Weight is OVER: Starting the Permanent Weight Loss Process

True weight loss and management is a process of restoring balance through individualizing your meals, which is unique for each person. The next step is to learn to eat from true physiological hunger and to stop when reaching satiation versus fullness or stomach pressure.

Eating from true "stomach" hunger can be difficult to learn and sometimes requires a very deliberate/conscious decision to clue-in to our bodies every time we pick up the fork (see *Listening to your Body chapter* for further help in this process).

This process is a journey and does become easier with practice. The process is learning the emotional cues connected to eating (anger, sadness, boredom, fatigue, guilt, fear, etc.). Frequently, emotions can well up during the course of the day leaving one in need of nurture or comfort. Eating can easily press down those feelings, by soothing or numbing them.

Learning to eat from internal vs. external cues is returning to "physically-connected" eating. [35] We've all heard messages like, "Clean the food on your plate," "Don't let this food go to waste," or "It's time for dinner now." These external cues often trigger eating past the point of satiation. We may not even be hungry when we begin a meal and only eat because the clock says it's time.

Eating from external cues keeps our weight above its natural state and size.

Dieting keeps us tied to the external state, dictating what is to be eaten and at what time intervals. Learning to connect to internal cues keeps us connected to our hunger. Examples that reinforce this may be: "I'm at a 2 on the hunger scale and it's only 11 a.m., but I need to eat lunch rather than waiting until noon when I may be at a 0;" or "It's dinner time, but I'm not that hungry and need to wait an hour or longer to eat so I will enjoy my meal."

Self Nurturing without Food and Setting Limits with Food

In her book called *The Solution*, Laurel Mellin, M.S., R.D. at UCSF Medical Center, talks about learning how to nurture oneself through the nurturing/limits cycle. [36] The nurturing cycle helps us work through our feelings and take care of them rather than eat them. The limiting cycle puts reasonable limits on our food selections so that we stay connected to our basic metabolism level.

This approach goes to the core of eating problems rather than masking the symptom of weight with a "diet fix." As part of healing our relationship with food forever, we can:

- Learn how to eat from physical hunger

- Honor our bodies when they tell us to stop

- Become aware of what emotional triggers we have developed over the years to help nurture and comfort ourselves

- Deal with our life problems, emotions, and feelings in ways other than turning to food.

Eating from internal cues takes time and is best done with the help of a registered dietitian who is knowledgeable in "hunger work."[35] Eating from true stomach hunger will begin the process of returning your body to its natural weight.

Maria's Story:
From Powerless to Powerful

When Maria came to see me she was overweight and in poor health. Together, we uncovered issues around her relationship with food, which she used to nurture herself through tough emotional times. This is her story:

I was a life-long, caretaking people pleaser weighing 331 pounds. My doctor had been warning me – though I wasn't diabetic YET, it would definitely be in my future if I didn't start making some healthy changes.

Historically, I did not have a weight problem until I went to college. After college I gained and lost the same 15-25 pounds through my 20s. In my 30s and 40s, I really started packing on the weight. I also had what I call an "early mid-life crisis" that sent me to therapy. Basically, I looked happy on the outside, but on the inside I was totally miserable.

As a result of therapy, I changed my life in ways that were positive, productive and just plain awesome. I left my unfulfilling job on Wall Street, became an Emmy-winning TV producer, came out of the closet, and fulfilled a dream moving from New York City to Los Angeles. But, I still struggled with my weight and was facing the same boring, exhausting challenges of food every day!

Enter God, fate, or whatever you want to call it. In 2007, I had orthopedic surgery and during the course of recovering, something happened to me. I don't know if I got scared by the thought of falling apart physically, or that I was no longer in my 20s. I began working out a lot. I joined a gym and met with a trainer for enough sessions to learn a good, manageable workout every day. It became the best, most favorite part of my day. This schedule continued for six months before I finally faced the fact that I wasn't losing weight due to my poor eating habits.

I decided I needed help educating myself about food and nutrition. Luckily, my brother had been seeing a nutritionist he'd been raving about. The first day I met Susan, my brother's dietitian, I changed my eating habits.

Over the next four months I lost about 50 pounds. I felt giddy. Susan was pleased, but didn't run down the path tossing rose petals and singing "Climb Every Mountain" with me. Instead, she was happy and supportive, but was quick to inform me that I was in the "honeymoon phase." She said it's a long haul and the core issue was still healing my relationship with food first.

Now, I am willing to look at what food does for me and am capable of seeing the real issues at hand that I was not willing to see before. To be clear, it's definitely an effort but it's no longer a struggle. Instead of feeling powerless like I have in the past, I now feel powerful. Being in touch with my real feelings makes life so much better. My mind is clear, and I'm healthy and happy!

Healing your relationship with food may be a mix of many different tools. This process does not happen overnight, but is well worth developing since the rewards are very satisfying.

Neal's Five Wonders

Neal is someone whose journey with weight hasn't been easy. In making a conscious choice to avoid the "diet trap" by adhering to a lifestyle process, Neal was able to successfully lose 80 pounds and maintain his target weight.

Neal came in for a nutrition consult 10 years ago due to insulin resistance and weight gain. He was referred by his physician. Neal speaks in his own words:

I love food. Food has been my source of comfort when I'm down, and it's the treat I give myself as a reward when I'm high. It is the way I soothe myself when I'm in an uncomfortable situation. Unfortunately my love affair with food was a classic case of an abusive relationship. In this instance however, I was both the abuser and the victim.

By the time I met Susan, I had lost control. I was 6'6", 300 lbs and I didn't see an end to my long history of problems with food. Susan was the first nutritionist who didn't put me on a diet. She worked with me to develop a plan that fit with my lifestyle, and in doing so, I changed my attitude and dependence on food.

Here are the five essential principles that

became totally necessary for me to lose weight. I glued these principles on my refrigerator, kept them on a business card in my wallet and tattooed them into my mind. It resulted in me saying 'goodbye' to 80 lbs, and I've managed to keep that weight off. Here's how I did it.

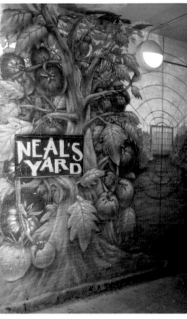

1) Practice environmental control: *It's hard enough to resist eating the bread they serve you before a meal at a restaurant, so don't put yourself through that torture at home. Make your home, office, any area you control -- a safe house for food. Get rid of EVERYTHING in your house that you shouldn't be eating! That includes sodas in the refrigerator, ice cream in the freezer, candy and sweets hidden in drawers or in your glovebox. If you don't see it, you won't be tempted to eat it. Fill your refrigerator, freezer and pantry with food you can eat: sliced lean meat, eggs, hard cheeses, nuts, fruits, salad ingredients and lots of vegetables.*

2) Exercise consistently: *This is my least favorite part, but I found that if you can keep your heart rate up for 45 minutes, four times a week you will accelerate the weight loss. You will feel more energized. You will get sick less often and most importantly, you will feel better about yourself! Running, brisk walking, stationary biking or aerobics are all good. Morning or night, as long as you break a sweat and devote 45 minutes to the effort.*

3) Eat in moderation: *I couldn't give up bread, ice cream or French fries. I just get too much pleasure out of them. I also knew they were the primary culprits in my weight gain. I made a deal with myself. I'd limit my consumption of my favorite foods to one day a week per food. And when I did eat them, I would cut my portion in half. When I got a sandwich, I'd only eat half the bread. When French fries were on my plate I'd eat only a few. When I had a scoop of ice cream, I'd limit my treat to one small scoop. Don't bother with the tofu bread, frozen yogurt or "air" French fries. Go for the real deal and enjoy it – but then move on after a small portion.*

4) Sleep: *The less sleep I got, the hungrier I was. Since I get up at 6 a.m. every morning for work, I forced myself (and all my friends and loved ones who ate with me) to eat an early dinner. Then I could be in bed by 10 p.m. Besides the savings you'll get from eating the "Early Bird Specials," the next day you'll be less susceptible to late night binge eating, and you'll feel focused and energized – ready to exercise again.*

5) Face the essential pain and focus on the rewards you are receiving: *Don't kid yourself. Changing your attitude toward food is going to hurt and will be challenging. In order to win the battle, you must come to terms with that fact. Although it might initially hurt to resist your favorite foods and reduce your portion size, the rewards you receive are more than worth the effort - weight loss, improved vitality, and a sense of well being. When I start to feel deprived, I remind myself of the changes I've made and how much better my life has become.*

Summary: So where does that leave us with the dieting process?

Since no easy fixes or solutions exist, try not to go on another quick fix diet or weight loss program. It can be a setup for failure and disappointment. The key takeaway here is that there is not one plan to lose weight quickly, keep it off, and move on with your life. Restoring health to your body requires going through the steps of individual needs, including medical issues, food choices to create balance, learning to eat from true physiological hunger, and exploring lifestyle factors that may be contributing to a weight issue. As we've seen from Maria's story and Neal's story, this is achievable!

Part Four

Nutrients Your Body Needs

Vitamins and Minerals: Food versus Pills

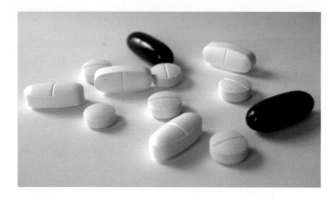

Do you ever get tired trying to figure out what food you need to eat in order to be healthy and energetic? Wouldn't it be easier to just take a pill, and eat whatever you have a craving for? From a statistical point of view, that is just what many Americans are doing. The Council for Responsible Nutrition in Washington, D.C. estimates that 64 percent of Americans are taking a vitamin/mineral supplement. According to the *Nutrition Business Journal*, sales of vitamins have risen steadily from $5 billion in 1995 to $10 billion in 2008.

How do we define a vitamin? A vitamin is an organic (meaning it contains carbon) substance that helps regulate essential functions within the cells of your body. There are 13 vitamins needed by humans, and they fall into the following two categories:

Water soluble (cannot be stored; need to be replenished)	Thiamin (vitamin B1) Riboflavin (vitamin B2) Niacin (vitamin B3) Folic acid B6 (pyridoxine) B12 Biotin Pantothenic acid Vitamin C
Fat soluble (stored in the liver or fat tissue)	Vitamin A Vitamin D Vitamin E Vitamin K

Minerals are inorganic substances. There are 2 classifications of minerals that exist: macro and trace. Macro-minerals are needed in amounts greater than 100 mg. and trace minerals are required in amounts less than 100 mg. They are as follows:

Macro-minerals (present in the body in large amounts)	Calcium Chloride Magnesium Phosphorus Potassium Sodium
Trace minerals (present in the body in smaller quantities)	Chromium Copper Fluoride Iodine Iron Manganese Molybdenum Selenium Zinc

RDAs: How Much Do You Really Need?

The Recommended Daily Allowances (**RDAs**) are published by the Food and Nutrition Board of the National Academy of Sciences (NAS) and are defined as the levels of needed nutrients "considered adequate to meet the known nutrient need of practically all healthy persons." The NAS establishes minimum amounts of vitamins and minerals necessary for most people living in the United States under usual environmental stresses and then adds a "safety margin" to that figure for possible additional needs. RDA values vary somewhat according to age and sex and are increased during pregnancy and lactation (breast-feeding). The NAS changes their recommendations on the RDA every few years depending on the current research.

Dietary Reference Intakes (**DRI**) are established by the Food and Nutrition Board of the National Academy of Sciences and Health Canada. These are a set of recommended intakes for nutrients for individuals according to their age and sex. A third set of numbers known as the Upper Intake Level (**UL**) is the level of a vitamin or mineral taken which would risk an adverse affect or toxicity level.

Most vitamin and mineral companies trying to get you to buy their supplements will say that the RDAs are outrageously low and that you need to take much more than the recommended amount.

Is it safe to take vitamins or minerals in large quantities? To answer this question practically, we need to look at the differences between water and fat-soluble vitamins, macro and trace minerals.

More specifics on the functions and food sources of vitamins and minerals can be found at the end of the chapter.

Water-Soluble vs. Fat-Soluble Vitamins

One of the most fundamental differences in a vitamin is whether it is **water-soluble** or **fat-soluble**. Water-soluble vitamins cannot be stored in the body for any great length of time, and therefore need to be frequently replenished via the diet. If large quantities of water-soluble vitamins are ingested, the body will use what it needs and the remainder will be excreted by the kidney into the urine. If the diet is low in water-soluble vitamins for several weeks to months, it is possible for a deficiency to develop. Many health professionals say that the body can safely handle almost any dose of water-soluble vitamins without posing any harmful side effects. However, a closer look at the research shows several water-soluble vitamins do have side effects at certain levels. It is important to know which vitamins act much like drugs and no longer function merely as nutrients when taken in large quantities.

Fat-soluble vitamins are not eliminated from the body when ingested in large quantities, but instead are stored in the liver and fat tissue. Several years of taking mega doses (defined as 5-10 times the RDA) of any fat-soluble vitamin can put you at possible risk for a toxicity.

How Do Vitamins Function in the Body?

Let's start with **vitamin C**, easily the most popular vitamin supplement. Also known by its chemical name, ascorbic acid, vitamin C is perhaps one of the most significant antioxidants that exists. To understand what an antioxidant is, we need to define what a free radical is. *Free radicals* are byproducts of normal reactions that happen within the body and can

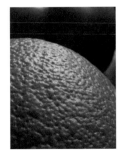

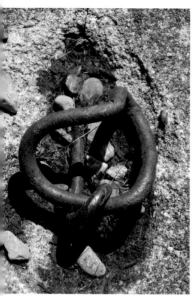

Oxidation is like rust

be produced by pollution or tobacco smoke. When free radicals are produced and are not "neutralized" or eliminated, they can damage your body's cells or result in what is known as oxidation (remember the apple turning brown or iron turning rusty?) Over time, an accumulation of free radicals in the body can contribute to heart disease, cancer, or premature aging. An antioxidant acts like a scavenger or fire extinguisher. It picks up free radicals, neutralizes them or rids the body of them, much like how lemon juice prevents an apple from browning.

Many scientists credit **vitamin C** with offering the body extra protection against cancer, heart disease, and cataracts. Additional roles of vitamin C, food sources, and RDA levels are found in the vitamin chart.

Individuals who eat 4-5 half-cup servings a day of vitamin C-rich foods have immune systems that are more effective at recognizing and fighting invading organisms from colds and the flu. Is meeting the RDA enough, or do you need to obtain mega-doses in the diet to meet your needs? Research to date doesn't justify amounts larger than 200-300 mg. of vitamin C per day, which can easily be met with a varied diet. (For comparison, consider that more than 250 mg. of vitamin C can be had by eating a small romaine lettuce salad with a tomato, some red bell pepper slices, and four strawberries.)

Vitamin C is a very important nutrient, but the amount recommended by some professionals and vitamin companies is probably excessive. Research shows that the maximum absorption of vitamin C in the tissues is about 250 mg. every four hours. So, if you're taking a 1,000 mg. tablet at one time, you will be excreting the rest in urine (thereby having very expensive urine!). Distortion of some medical tests is another side effect of high vitamin C supplementation. For example, when testing the blood for cholesterol levels, taking vitamin C supplements may distort the accuracy of the test.

Nobel Prize winner Linus Pauling was one of the first scientists who touted vitamin C as the latest miracle of the '70s and '80s, curing everything from the basic cold to cancer.

Double-blind studies (ones where neither the researchers nor the participants knew what they were receiving) found that taking vitamin C did not prevent colds, but did help in alleviating some of the symptoms, since high doses of C act like an antihistamine (remember that large doses of vitamins act like drugs). People report feeling better from colds after taking vitamin C, but what they are really feeling is the antihistamine effect of vitamin C, which occurs in levels above 250 mg. They still have the cold, but taking a lot of vitamin C can mask the symptoms much like common antihistamines like Sudafed™ do.

It is not clearly known whether vitamin C prevents disease. Research to date shows conflicting results whether increased amounts of vitamin C lowers risk of heart disease, cancer or other medical issues.

Are there any side effects of too much or not enough vitamin C?

Vitamin C deficiency eventually leads to *scurvy*, a weakening of collagen in the body, which can lead to bleeding. Excess vitamin C can also cause problems. Some people who take large amounts of vitamin C (e.g. over 1,000 mg.) can be at an increased risk for kidney stones, specifically calcium-oxalate stones. Taking 1,000-4,000 mg. of vitamin C per day can increase oxalate (a chemical substance) excretion in the body since vitamin C is a precursor of oxalate.

Other potential side effects include cramping and diarrhea when taking levels of vitamin C over 500-1,000 mg. Overall, vitamin C is very important to your health, but large amounts of this vitamin need to be taken with caution.

Several clients recently consulted me for nutritional counseling due to severe gastrointestinal problems such as cramping and diarrhea. After looking at their diets and supplement histories, it became apparent that most of their symptoms began shortly after starting 1,000-4,000 mg. per day of vitamin C supplements. After stopping the vitamin C, all cramping and diarrhea stopped with no reoccurrence of symptoms.

In addition, I cannot count the number of clients who come to me for advice regarding a diet to prevent kidney stones. All of these clients have been taking over 1,000 mg. per day of vitamin C. Upon discontinuing the vitamin C, none had a reoccurrence of stones. When self-prescribing vitamins, it is important to look at your vitamin intake and see if the vitamins are causing, or have the potential of causing, any physical problems.

And Now for the B's

B vitamins are essential for conversion of food into energy. Contrary to popular belief, vitamins do not supply energy, but aid in reactions converting food to energy. For details on the roles and food sources of vitamins, refer to the vitamin chart at the end of the chapter. **Vitamin B1 (Thiamin)** deficiency is rare in the United States, but symptoms of

deficiency include fatigue, weakness, and nerve damage. **Vitamin B2 (Riboflavin)** deficiency is also uncommon, but is manifested with dry, flaky skin and eye disorders. Toxicity is rarely seen in either vitamin.

Niacin (Vitamin B3) deficiency is rare except in those who don't consume adequate protein in their diets. This can result in a condition known as *pellagra*, which is characterized by diarrhea, mental impairment, and digestive problems. Pellagra is relatively rare now, but at the turn of the century it was fairly common in the American South, where the diet of the poor was fairly low in protein.

Mega doses of niacin (doses exceeding 300 mg./day) can be dangerous and cause rashes, nausea, diarrhea, and liver damage. Niacin is sometimes therapeutically prescribed to lower cholesterol levels, but should be done under the supervision of a physician, since high doses of niacin are irritating to the liver.

Vitamin B6 (pyridoxine) deficiency is uncommon, but can cause mental convulsions in infants. High doses of B6 have been advocated to treat symptoms of premenstrual syndrome (PMS). Mega doses (over 100 mg./day) have been known to cause a condition known as *peripheral neuritis*. The symptoms of peripheral neuritis are similar to multiple sclerosis, which includes numbness and tingling in the hands, difficulty walking, and pain in the spine.

Folic acid is especially important during pregnancy. Studies have shown that folic acid supplementation is associated with a reduction of neural tube defects and *Spina Bifida* (one type of defect in the neural tube which becomes the spinal cord of the baby). Deficiency is rare, since folic acid is plentiful in a variety of foods, but can result in anemia or birth defects.

Consuming too much folic acid can mask a vitamin B12 deficiency. Until recently, it was recommended that additional folic acid be taken to lower rates of heart disease. However, current studies show folic acid may actually increase cardiovascular risk, and therefore it is recommended that only woman of child bearing age take a folic acid supplement.

When it comes to folic acid, most multivitamin supplements contain the RDA of 400 micrograms per day. Recent studies have linked excess folic acid with an increased risk of colorectal, breast and prostate cancers. Therefore, the recommendation is to take a multivitamin mineral supplement every other day, or 3-4 times per week, since you will most likely be getting folic acid in the foods that you consume as well (unless you are pregnant or of child-bearing age).

Vitamin B12 (cyanocobalamin) is produced from bacteria in the gut and is present in foods or animals which have ingested the bacteria. Therefore, vitamin B12 is only present in animal products. Symptoms of B12 deficiency include fatigue, anemia, and nerve damage. Some people can become B12 deficient by lacking a substance produced in the stomach lining called *intrinsic factor* that aids in absorbing B12. This deficiency is known as *pernicious anemia*, but is quite rare.

A common phenomenon in older individuals is a B12 deficiency due to an inadequate amount of stomach acids, since stomach acids are required to release B12 from the food source. A University of Oxford study done in 2007 showed that increased levels of B12 may reduce the rate of age-related cognitive decline and dementia by 30 percent. Additionally, older individuals should maximize foods that are good sources of B12 in addition to taking a supplement. There are no known manifestations of taking excess amounts of vitamin B12.

Many people receive B12 supplements on the premise that they are lacking in energy. However, B12 does not supply energy, and rarely does one see a deficiency except in vegans (those consuming no animal, egg or dairy products) or vegetarians who are not vigilant about consuming adequate protein.

It has been shown that B12 shots can provide an analgesic effect, which means they can make you feel good. According to Julie Sease, PharmD, clinical assistant professor at South Carolina College of Pharmacy, there is little available information on the use of treating fatigue with B12 shots in those without a deficiency.[37] She recommends further investigation be done to show proof that the treatment of fatigue with B12 shots is beneficial, since the few studies to date do not show fatigue is lowered.

The last two water-soluble vitamins are **pantothenic acid** and **biotin**. Deficiency or toxicity is rarely seen in either vitamin – see the chart for more details.

Fat-soluble Vitamins – A, E, D, K

Vitamin A is present in foods in one form called *retinol*, but it can also be formed in the body from its carotenoid form, *beta-carotene*, an antioxidant that will be covered in the *Phytochemical* chapter. Vitamin A deficiency can cause vision problems such as night blindness, dry, scaly skin, and problems with reproduction. Vitamin A toxicity is not uncommon, since it cannot be excreted, and is therefore stored in the body. Symptoms of toxicity include: irreversible liver damage, abnormal development of a fetus, headaches, bone pain, skin changes, vomiting, loss of appetite, loss of hair, and nerve damage.

Most of the time, a toxicity results from over-supplementation and not from excess food intake.

One client who had been taking large doses of vitamin A had all her hair fall out and was extremely sick for many weeks. Fortunately, she had no lasting effects, but there are reported cases of death from toxicity of this vitamin. It is recommended that pregnant women take less vitamin A than the RDA and not consume foods that are fortified with extra vitamin A since it can cause birth defects.

Vitamin E (also known as tocopherol) was a highly recommended antioxidant supplement until recent research found that those who take regular high-dose vitamin E supplements may increase their risk of mortality. There is some evidence that taking extra vitamin E may be problematic for people who have blood-clotting issues. If these same patients are taking anticoagulant drugs, like Coumadin®, vitamin E may increase the risk for a bleeding-related stroke. Vitamin E deficiency is rare, except with people who have problems absorbing fat.

Vitamin K assists with proper blood clotting. Deficiency is rare since our body is able to make most of the vitamin K we need from the bacteria in our intestines, with the rest supplied by our diets. Deficiency can be present when people cannot absorb vitamin K or are taking excessive antibiotics that kill off the gut bacteria that produce this vitamin. Some infants lack the bacteria that make vitamin K. A toxicity of vitamin K has not been observed. People who are taking blood-thinning agents need to avoid large amounts of high vitamin K foods, since they interact with these medications.

Vitamin D is also known as the "sunshine vitamin," and its deficiency can lead to rickets or soft bones in children. In adults, the risk of deficiency is *osteomalacia* (softening of the bone) or *osteoporosis* (bone loss). Vitamin D facilitates calcium absorption and promotes bone mineralization.

Many health care professionals are now touting it

as a protection against many forms of disease. A great way to get your vitamin D, besides food, is exposure to daylight or sunshine three times per week for about 10-15 minutes, since your skin has the ability to manufacture it after being exposed to sunlight. Since many of us try to stay out of sun due to skin cancer, we are deficient in natural vitamin D.

Until very recently, it was thought that the RDA for vitamin D (400 IU/day) was sufficient to prevent disease and to maintain bone health. We have recently seen an epidemic of vitamin D deficiency in the U.S., which is thought to be responsible for many autoimmune diseases, such as rheumatoid arthritis and Multiple Sclerosis, cancers and even cardiovascular disease.

What are the recent findings on Vitamin D?[38]

- A 2007 analysis of 18 studies published in the *Archives of Internal Medicine* found *cholecalciferol* (also known as vitamin D3) significantly reduced mortality [39]

- Vitamin D deficiency is highly associated with cardiac disease, high blood pressure, stroke, diabetes, mental illness and chronic pain

- Taking 2,000 IU of vitamin D per day for one year virtually eliminated self-reported incidences of colds and flus [39]

- A Canadian endocrinology clinic that gave their patients 4,000 IU of vitamin D per day for six months showed no side effects other than improved mood

- Pregnant and lactating women may need as much as 5,000-10,000 IU/day

- Too much vitamin A antagonizes the action of vitamin D and can negate its protective effect

Benefits of vitamin D are more important than we all knew – lowering risk of death, many diseases, colds, and flus.

Some researchers are now calling vitamin D "the antibiotic vitamin," since it boosts protection in the white blood cells of antimicrobial compounds that defend the body against germs.[40] Many physicians are recommending 1,000-2,000 IU of vitamin D per day to help with already low blood levels to help prevent disease (*see osteoporosis section of book*).

Minerals

Macro-Minerals

Sodium, **chloride** and **potassium** are macro-minerals, as well as being major electrolytes. The body requires at least 500 mg. of sodium per day, which is easily achieved with a normal diet. Potassium is a very important electrolyte needed by the body and is widely available in many foods. Surprisingly, many people take expensive potassium supplements when it is easy to obtain more than enough potassium simply with a general diet.

Phosphorus aids in building strong bones and teeth along with **calcium** and **magnesium**. Magnesium is important in the function of nerves, bones and muscles. Nausea, weakness, muscular weakness, and spasms are some of the effects of magnesium deficiency. Low intakes of magnesium are linked to high blood pressure, heart abnormalities, or cardiac arrest. Deficiencies are not common unless you are taking diuretics or have prolonged vomiting or diarrhea. Magnesium toxicity is uncommon, except in those with kidney

disease, or if a person is taking large doses of magnesium containing supplements or drugs.

Calcium is critical in the body, and it's surprising how little we get of it. With the major "fat phobia" common in our culture, many Americans (especially adolescents) have heard to "cut down on dairy," and have done so accordingly. However, there are many low fat dairy foods available, and the calcium they provide is essential to building and maintaining strong bones and teeth.

Besides its major role in prevention of osteoporosis, several important research studies have shown that calcium can assist with lowering blood pressure.

There has been a lot of attention on the relationship between calcium and weight management. The studies are trying to establish how this works, but it appears that **calcium in food stimulates fat breakdown**. If you increase your intake of dietary calcium along with a normal protein intake, there is an increase of fat in your stool and an increase in energy metabolism by as much as 350 calories per day. It seems that when there is a higher level of calcium within the cells of the body, less fat is deposited in those cells. The studies also showed low calcium diets increased the level of fat storage. This phenomenon has not been observed with calcium supplements.

Optimal intakes of calcium for women are 1,200-1,500 mg. depending on age, pregnancy or post-menopausal years. For men, the recommended intake is 1,000 mg. per day.

If calcium intake is a problem for you due to *lactose intolerance* (the inability to break down the sugar in milk resulting in bloating, gas or diarrhea), calcium supplements may be a good option. If you have lactose intolerance, there are excellent lactose-reduced milk products and pills you can drop into milk to help break down the indigestible sugar lactose, assisting your body with tolerance to dairy products. Due to varying levels of lactose intolerance, some people can eat small amounts of cheese or yogurt, since about 90-95 percent of the lactose has been broken down.

If calcium supplements are required due to severe lactose intolerance, it is important to differentiate between the different types of calcium supplements. Calcium citrate, carbonate, gluconate, lactate, dolomite, and bone meal are all types of calcium supplements. Calcium citrate or carbonate are the most absorbable forms of calcium and are readily available. **Be sure to avoid calcium supplements with dolomite or bone meal since they may contain small amounts of lead, aluminum or other metals that can lead to dangerous levels in the blood or toxicity.** If you are taking iron supplements, take them at different times than the calcium supplements for the best absorption.

One common side effect of calcium supplementation is constipation, so be sure to drink plenty of water if you are supplementing with calcium. Of course, food is always the best option over supplements since the calcium in food is better absorbed in amounts the body can readily use and take in. In addition, it is questionable exactly how much of a supplement is actually absorbed. However, with severe lactose intolerance, supplements are a good option, in addition to other non-dairy sources of calcium, such as green leafy vegetables.

Are there any unfavorable effects of too much supplemental calcium? Intake of calcium supplements above 2,500 mg. has been associated with decreased absorption of zinc, iron, and other essential minerals as well as constipation.

Trace Minerals

Iron is a trace mineral essential in helping form the oxygen carrier in your red blood cells called *hemoglobin*, and the oxygen carrier in your muscles called *myoglobin*. There are two types of iron:

- *heme*, found in meat and animal products

- *nonheme*, found in plant-based foods

Heme iron is much more absorbable by the body than non-heme iron. If iron is lacking in your diet, the red blood cells cannot carry as much oxygen to the tissues. This may result in fatigue, weakness, or lack of energy, also known as anemia. Periods in life that may require larger amounts of iron:

- childhood

- adolescence

- child-bearing years for women, since they have monthly blood losses

- pregnancy

- elderly years, when diets often lack iron-rich foods

Various factors help influence how well iron is absorbed. The absorption rate of heme iron is normally between 15-30 percent. On the whole, nonheme iron absorption varies as much as tenfold, or between 2-20 percent. What increases or decreases the absorption?

Vitamin C and foods containing vitamin C *increase* the absorption of iron in nonheme iron foods.

Calcium phosphate, **oxalates** in spinach and chocolate, **phytates** in wheat and unfermented soy products and legumes, **polyphenols** in coffee and tea, **tannins** in tea, and **antacids** can significantly _decrease_ nonheme iron absorption.

Another way to boost absorption of nonheme iron is to consume it with a food containing heme iron. So, if you're eating a piece of lean meat for dinner (heme iron), have a spinach salad (nonheme iron) to enhance the absorption of iron in the spinach.

Iron supplements or high-iron foods need to be avoided by some groups of people. A group of Finnish researchers in 1992 reported that men who had medium to high blood iron levels were more likely to develop heart disease than those with low to normal blood iron levels.

Since that time, some researchers have associated increased amounts of iron with free radical formation, which in turn can increase the risk of atherosclerosis and cardiovascular disease. Therefore, it is not recommended that a person start taking iron supplements unless under a physician's supervision due to a diagnosed iron-deficiency anemia. Taking iron supplements without a need can interfere with absorption of other minerals in the body such as calcium and zinc since they have similar receptor sites in your cells.

Chromium has received a lot of attention in the last 20 years. Chromium deficiency is rare in this country and hard to diagnose. If a true deficiency exists, it can look like diabetes (i.e. higher blood sugars). However, few diabetics have been helped by chromium supplementation.

Some studies done in China found that large doses of chromium picolinate were helpful in controlling blood sugar. However, the Chinese diet is vastly different than the U.S. diet, and the study has not been duplicated in the U.S. Fortunately, in 1996, the Federal Trade Commission (FTC) forced three of the leading marketers of chromium picolinate

to stop making claims that chromium assisted with weight loss, building muscle, burning fat, lowering cholesterol or blood glucose levels since there were no studies that substantiated these claims. Chromium toxicity is extremely rare from dietary sources, and it is unknown at this point if there is any risk of toxicity from supplementation. In looking at countless studies done on varying levels of chromium supplementation, no conclusive benefits have been demonstrated.

Selenium works as an antioxidant along with vitamin E to protect cells from damage or oxidation that can lead to diseases such as cancer, heart disease or premature aging. A study published in the _Journal of the American Medical Association_ in 1996 studied 1,300 people who previously had skin cancer to see if taking a daily selenium supplement prevented the reoccurrence of skin cancer.[41] The supplements had no effect on skin cancer, but total cancer incidence and mortality of lung, prostrate and colon cancer were roughly cut by half, which was a big surprise to the researchers. One of the limitations of the study was that it was done in the Southeastern area of the U.S. where people don't receive as much selenium from their food because it is grown in selenium-poor soil. Other parts of the country might not have had such a dramatic effect on lowering cancer rates.

Selenium deficiency is rare in humans. Selenium can be quite toxic in high doses (amounts greater than 200 mcg. /day) with symptoms of nervous system damage, hair and nail loss, nausea, abdominal pain, diarrhea, fatigue and irritability.

Zinc has some basic functions, which can be found in the mineral chart; additionally, it is involved in activating vitamin A in the retina to prevent night blindness, as well as maintaining healthy skin, hair, nails, and healing wounds. The zinc found in animal protein is much more readily available than that found in vegetable sources. The latter contain *phytic* acid, which can bind with zinc, making it less available for absorption.

Zinc deficiency is rare, but people at risk are:

- Heavy drinkers (alcohol speeds up zinc excretion)

- Those with gastrointestinal diseases (lowers absorption in the gut)

- Restrained eaters, such as those with anorexia nervosa, who have chronically poor intakes of calories and protein

- Vegans (those who eat no animal, egg or dairy products) and those who consume low amounts of protein

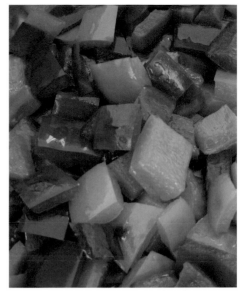

Red and orange peppers: packed with vitamin C and carotenoids

Symptoms of deficiency include: appetite loss, taste changes, skin changes, delayed wound healing and less resistance to infection. What about too much zinc? Taking mega doses of zinc can interfere with the body's absorption of copper. Mega doses of zinc can depress the immune system and interfere with the body's ability to form red blood cells. In addition, HDL cholesterol (remember the happy cholesterol?) can be reduced significantly with zinc supplementation, thereby raising the risk for heart disease.

You may have heard about using zinc to treat a cold. A study done in 1996 at the Cleveland Clinic tested zinc gluconate lozenges on 99 people to see what the effect on a cold would be. [42] Half the group received the zinc gluconate lozenges and the other half received placebo lozenges every two hours for the first 24 hours of the cold. It was found that the zinc takers' cold symptoms cleared up about three days sooner than the placebo group.

However, a large percentage of the zinc group complained of a bad mouth taste and nausea - maybe not such a great tradeoff for a few more days of blowing your nose!

The other five trace minerals — **copper, iodine, fluoride, manganese, and molybdenum** — have important functions, but a deficiency or toxicity is rarely seen. Refer to the table on minerals for a list of roles and food sources for each of these minerals.

Micronutrients Over Time

After hearing all about vitamins and minerals, what is the bottom line? Many individuals do not need a vitamin and mineral supplement, even if their diet is not optimal.

Individuals lacking in energy usually need to alter their macronutrient intake (i.e. carbohydrate, protein, and fat) rather than their micronutrient intake (i.e. vitamins and minerals).

It is important to think of the food you eat in terms of a week's time rather than a day. For example, if you have a variety of foods over a week, meeting more of the RDA for one nutrient on one day and less on another day, your body will take that into account and make up for it. You do not have to meet the RDA for every vitamin and mineral every day – look at what you eat over the course of a week.

There are four major reasons why people need a supplement (besides those outlined in the alternate list below):

- Chronically low calorie intake (below 1,500 calories) making it difficult to receive adequate nutrients

- Extremely poor food choices - no fruits and vegetables and reliance on processed foods only

- Substance abuse such as alcohol or drugs

- Having a specific disease that make it difficult to absorb or receive adequate nutrients via the diet, such Crohn's disease, colitis or in the case of burn patients

Who may need a vitamin and mineral supplement?

- **Children** under the age of four when the body is first developing

- **Women of childbearing age**: it is well-established that folic acid supplementation is important for preventing birth defects. Extra iron may be necessary for those with heavy menstrual cycles and during pregnancy and lactation. Calcium may be important during pregnancy and lactation since it will be taken from the mother if not supplied in adequate amounts in the diet

- **Older adults**: women may need additional calcium, especially if they are not on hormone replacement therapy, for prevention of osteoporosis. Vitamin D may be necessary and levels should be checked for both men and women. In addition, Vitamin B12 may be necessary due to poor absorption

- **Vegetarians**: specifically vegans who consume no dairy or egg products who are at risk for vitamin B12 deficiency, as well as some of the minerals

- **Smokers and alcoholics**: studies have shown that smokers have lower levels of vitamin A, C and E in their blood and may benefit from a supplement. Those with large intakes of alcohol may consume a majority of their calories as alcohol. In addition, deficiency of some of the B vitamins is possible, since alcohol interferes with the metabolism of B vitamins

Buying Supplements

If you are taking a supplement for "insurance purposes," it's best to choose one that is balanced with respect to all the various vitamins and minerals and has less or equal to 100 percent of the RDA for most things. A good Web site is Consumerlab.com, which evaluates supplements and tells you whether they actually contain what the label states, and if they are of good quality.

There are small differences between "natural" and "synthetic" vitamins and minerals except for the price. Rather than buying a brand name, it might be just as beneficial to buy a generic drug-store type for economical purposes. If a vitamin supplement were truly "natural," it would cost so much that no one could afford to buy it! Some of the lesser expensive supplements do contain fillers, or substances that are not needed in the supplement, so make sure to check the label.

Also, check the expiration date on the label since vitamins (just like drugs) lose their potency after a certain amount of time. Fish oil supplements need to be properly stored since they can go rancid, so buying a quality brand of this supplement is essential. Being educated about the amounts of vitamins or minerals in the supplements you are taking is important since taking too much of one vitamin or mineral may interfere with the absorption of another.

Many supplement companies are seductive in the way they introduce and sell their vitamins to the public. Common gimmicks are "timed-released" vitamins which in studies only lasted two hours compared with the claims of lasting six to eight hours. Many recent companies state their minerals are different since they are "chelated," which means they have gone through a process where the mineral is bonded with a protein to enhance its absorption into the cells of the body. They enhance absorption, but no research to date has shown enhanced retention within the cells of the body with chelated minerals.

Summary

Why consume a variety of foods rather than popping a pill? Research has shown that although foods have identifiable vitamins and minerals, they contain many non-vitamin and mineral substances that assist in disease prevention and cannot be duplicated in a pill. The next chapter will focus on these non-vitamin and mineral substances called phytochemicals. In addition, foods contain nutrients in amounts the body needs and can readily utilize.

When you think of supplements, think about them by definition: things you take to supplement an already healthy diet full of nutrient dense foods, and not something you take as a substitute when consuming an unhealthy diet.

Chart on Vitamins

Vitamins	Role in Health	RDA/DRI	Best Food Sources	Example of Foods to meet RDA
Water-Soluble				
Vitamin C (Ascorbic Acid)	Wound healing, formation and repair of connective tissue, role in healthy gums and teeth, potent antioxidant	60-90 mg.	Citrus fruits and juices, berries, kiwis, papayas, melons, kale, tomatoes, broccoli, cauliflower, sweet potatoes, peppers	One medium orange
Vitamin B1 (Thiamin)	Carbohydrate metabolism, necessary for healthy nervous system and heart function	1.1-1.5 mg.	Lean meat, pork, seeds, legumes	3 oz. of lean broiled sirloin steak
Vitamin B2 (Riboflavin)	Carbohydrate metabolism, involved with red blood cell function, healthy skin and eyes	1.1-1.5 mg.	Dairy products, lean meat, eggs, green leafy vegetables, beans, fruit	Two cups of milk and one cup of blueberries
Vitamin B3 (Niacin)	Metabolism of carbohydrate, fat, and protein into energy	14-20 mg.	Lean meat, poultry, fish, eggs, nuts, dairy products, mushrooms, peanuts	One roasted chicken breast, 2 tbsp. of peanut butter and 5 small mushrooms
Vitamin B6 (Pyridoxine)	Protein metabolism, maintains normal brain function, aids in formation of red blood cells	1.3-2.0 mg.	Lean meat, fish, nuts, lentils, bananas, cauliflower, chicken, eggs, avocados	One banana, four ounce piece of fish and a handful of sunflower seeds
Folic Acid	Works with vitamin B12 to form red blood cells, needed to make DNA, RNA (genetic part of cells)	200-400 mcg.	Dark green leafy vegetables, citrus fruits, sunflower seeds, legumes	One cup of cooked spinach and one medium papaya
Vitamin B12 (Cyanocobalamin)	Needed to make red blood cells, DNA, RNA, and the myelin shealth (protects nerve fibers)	2.0-2.4 mcg.	Meat, poultry, fish, eggs, milk, and other dairy products	Four ounce piece of fish or lean meat

Vitamins	Role in Health	RDA/DRI	Best Food Sources	Example of Foods to meet RDA
Water-Soluble				
Pantothenic Acid	Carbohydrate, protein and fat metabolism	5 mg.	Mushrooms, sunflower seeds, yogurt, broccoli, winter squash and eggs	One cup of mushrooms, an egg and a handful of sunflower seeds
Biotin	Carbohydrate, protein and fat metabolism	30 mcg.	Eggs, ricotta cheese, cheese, peanut butter	2 tablespoons of peanut butter
Fat-Soluble				
Vitamin A	Promotes good vision, prevents night blindness, maintains healthy skin, teeth and tissues in the mouth, stomach and intestines	700-900 mcg.	Eggs, liver, cod liver oil, milk, dark green leafy vegetables, yellow or orange fruits and vegetables	½ a cantaloupe or ½ cup of butternut squash
Vitamin D	Promotes absorption of calcium and phosphorus in the body, builds and maintains strong bones and teeth	400 IU	Milk, eggs, butter, fatty fish with bones	4 oz. of canned salmon
Vitamin E	Prevention of heart disease, cataracts and cancer, improves immunity, antioxidant	15 mg.	Poultry, nuts, seeds, fish, eggs	¼ cup of almonds
Vitamin K	Blood clotting	90-120 mcg.	Spinach, broccoli, cabbage, eggs	½ cup of broccoli

mg. = milligrams
mcg. = micrograms

Chart on Minerals

Minerals	Role in Health	RDA/DRI	Best Food Sources	Example of Foods to meet RDA
Macro-Minerals				
Sodium	Electrolyte that regulates water balance and blood pressure, transmits nerve signals	500 mg.	Salt	¼ teaspoon of salt
Chloride	Electrolyte that regulates fluid balance, used to make digestive juices	750 mg.	Salt, seafood	¼ teaspoon of salt
Potassium	Electrolyte that helps regulate fluid balance with sodium, aids in muscle contraction, nerve impulses, heart, kidney function	2000-4700 mg.	Oranges, bananas, avocados, tomatoes, milk, yogurt, nuts, papaya	One avocado, one banana, and ¼ cup of almonds
Phosphorus	Important in energy metabolism,helps maintain strong bones and teeth	700-1200 mg.	Meat, poultry, milk products, nuts, seeds, eggs	2 oz.of Swiss cheese and a handful of sunflower seeds
Magnesium	Important in function of nerves, bones, and muscles, aids in normal heart rhythm	80-400 mg.	Nuts, beans, bananas, dark green vegetables, dark chocolate	Handful of almonds and a small piece of dark chocolate
Calcium	Builds strong bones and teeth, necessary for regulating heart-beat, aids in blood clotting	800-1200 mg.	Milk, plain yogurt, ricotta cheese, cheese	One cup of plain yogurt, and ¾ cup of ricotta cheese

Minerals	Role in Health	RDA/DRI	Best Food Sources	Example of Foods to meet RDA
Trace-Minerals				
		Males		
Iron	Helps form hemoglobin (oxygen carrier in the blood) and myoglobin (oxygen carrier in muscle)	10-15 mg.	Lean red meats, fish, poultry, legumes, nuts and seeds	4 oz. piece of lean red meat and ¼ cup of pumpkin seeds
Chromium	Works with insulin to assist in glucose (sugar) metabolism	50-200 mcg.	Mushrooms, onions, melon, papaya, nuts	One papaya
Selenium	Antioxidant along with vitamin E to protect cells from damage or oxidation leading to disease	55-70 mcg.	Fish, shellfish, red meat, eggs, chicken, brazil nuts	5 oz. piece of salmon
Zinc	Growth and repair of all cells, maintains normal appetite and taste perception, immunity, sexual maturation	10-15 mg.	Seafood (especially oysters) red meat, eggs, legumes	One steamed oyster
Copper	Aids in forming red blood cells	900 mcg.	Meat, seafood, nuts and seeds	¼ cup of sunflower seeds
Iodine	Important in thyroid metabolism	150 mcg.	Iodized salt, milk products	1½ cups of milk and 2 eggs
Fluoride	Aids in forming bones and teeth	2-4 mg.	Fluoridated water, fish, tea	6 oz. of cooked cod
Manganese	Assists with energy production	1.8-2.3 mg.	Coconut, nuts, peanut butter, berries	2 tbsp. of peanut butter and 1 tbsp. of pecans
Molybdenum	Part of many enzymes in the body	45 mcg.	Buckwheat, eggs, beans, cabbage, spinach	2 tbsp. of cooked beans

Phytochemicals

If you want to lower your risk of cancer or heart disease AND increase your immune function, you need to know the basics about phytochemicals.

Phytochemicals, also known as **phytonutrients**, are substances that plants naturally contain to protect themselves against sunlight, bacteria or viruses and oxidation – kind of like a natural sunscreen. Simply put, once we *eat* these plants, our immunity increases, and we become more resistant to cancer, heart disease and other medical problems.

It is estimated that there may be well over 100 phytochemicals in one serving of a fruit or vegetable. That is potentially as many as 13,000 different phytonutrients in our food supply! Each day brings the discovery of more types, and more information about how phytonutrients work. Because of the concentration of nutrients, you can see how easy it is to increase your health by adding just one extra serving of fruit or vegetable per day.

Phytochemicals have many antioxidant properties, and each of them work in the body in a unique way.

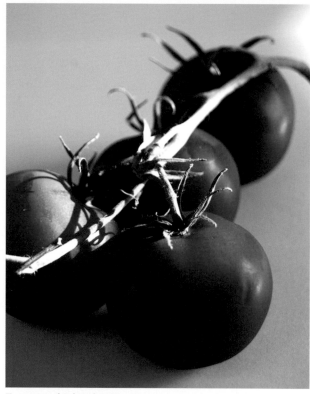

Tomatoes: high in lycopenes

There are many other categories, but let's focus on three key ones presently highlighted by researchers that have antioxidant activitity.

- carotenoids
- polyphenols (including flavonoids)
- thiosulfonates

PHYTOCHEMICALS / PHYTONUTRIENTS

CAROTENOIDS

LYCOPENES
- Guavas
- Tomatoes
- Tomato Products
- Watermelon

LUTEIN
- Avocado
- Egg Yolks
- Kale
- Spinach

ZEAXANTHIN
- Brussels Sprouts
- Kale
- Romaine Lettuce
- Zucchini

BETA-CAROTENE
- Apricots
- Cantaloupe
- Carrots
- Collard Greens
- Pumpkin
- Spinach
- Sweet Potatoes

ALPHA-CAROTENE
- Cantaloupe
- Carrots
- Guava
- Pumpkin

POLYPHENOLS

FLAVONOIDS

QUERCETIN
- Apples
- Buckwheat
- Green Tea
- Red Grapes

ANTHOCYANINS
- Blackberries
- Blueberries
- Green Tea
- Raspberries

CATECHINS/EPICATECHINS
- Dark Chocolate
- Green Tea
- White Tea

NON-FLAVONOIDS

RESVERATROL
- Black Tea
- Grape Skins
- Green Tea

LIGNANS
- Ground Flaxseeds
- Walnuts

CURCUMIN
- Turmeric

THIOSULFONATES

ALLYLLIC SULFIDES (Alliums)
- Garlic
- Leeks
- Onions
- Shallots

Category 1: Carotenoids

Carotenoids are the most well known group of phytochemicals. Scientists have discovered approximately 600 different carotenoids. Carotenoids play a role in the prevention of cancer, heart disease, and maintaining healthy eyes. Most of us have heard of beta-carotene, but there are a host of other carotenoids such as lycopenes, lutein, zeaxanthin, and alpha-carotene.

- **Lycopenes**, or the red carotenoids, are found in tomatoes and tomato products, watermelon, guava, and pink grapefruit, and have been found to be helpful in preventing prostate cancer. A 1997 Harvard study showed that men who ate tomatoes or tomato products (10 or more servings per week) had a 35 percent lowered risk of prostate cancer. Similar studies have not shown as great an effect.

- **Lutein**: found in green leafy vegetables such as kale, spinach, avocado and in egg yolks, lutein is helpful for maintaining eye health. Lutein in egg yolks is a yellow carotenoid.

- **Zeaxanthin**: considered the sister to lutein, it is found in kale, romaine lettuce, Brussels sprouts and zucchini. Studies show that it is helpful in the prevention of age-related macular degeneration.

- **Beta and Alpha Carotene**: (the orange carotenoids) beta-carotene, which is converted to vitamin A as the body requires it, is found in sweet potatoes, carrots, apricots, spinach, collard greens, pumpkin and cantaloupe. Alpha-carotene is found in similar foods such as pumpkin, carrots, cantaloupe, and guava. There has been an association between high beta carotene levels in the blood and lower incidence of lung cancer (via the diet and not with supplements).

A carrot can contain as many as 100 different carotenoids, whereas a beta carotene supplement has only one type of beta carotene, demonstrating the benefits of consuming food versus taking a vitamin. Furthermore, you receive the benefit of the fiber and fullness of the actual food when you eat the carrot.

Category 2: Polyphenols

Polyphenols are the new hot topic you see in research studies and in many magazines. There are two additional categories (see the chart for clarification). One category of Polyphenols has a class of pigments called **flavonoids**. Flavonoids, also known as bioflavonoids, have antioxidant activity and are known for their prevention of heart disease and cancer, since they can lower cholesterol levels and inflammatory processes in the body.

Three common **flavonoids** are:

- **Quercetin:** found in the greatest concentration in apple skins

- **Anthocyanins**: present in the patriotic red, blue and purple fruits; the highest concentration is in berries

- **Catechins**: present in tea (specifically green and white) and epicatechins found in cocoa (major ingredient in dark chocolate)

What are some great ways to add these foods to your everyday diet?

- Enjoy an apple with peanut butter in the afternoon, or cut up a few apple slices and serve in your evening salad

- For a healthy breakfast, add a variety of brightly colored berries on your cottage cheese, ricotta cheese or plain yogurt

- Melt ½ ounce of greater than 70 percent dark chocolate in your milk at night for healthy hot cocoa

- Substitute your morning coffee with green tea

The quercetin in apples is thought to lower LDL (remember the lousy?) cholesterol and decrease plaque in the arteries. Apples also contain pectin, a type of fiber which can lower cholesterol.

Extensive research by food scientist Rui Hai Liu from Cornell University in June 2007 found apples have substances that fight cancer cells and reduce the number and size of tumors in rats. [43] He also discovered that apples contain another compound known as *triterpeniods* in the peel, which can inhibit or kill cancer cells.

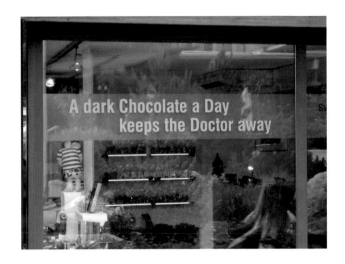

Benefits of the whole apple

Eat the entire apple, since the key nutrients are in the peel and the interior. Organic are preferred since apples are one of the fruits having the highest amount of pesticides. The old adage of "an apple a day keeps the doctor away" may be more apropos than we moderns first realized.

The anthocyanins making berries red, blue and purple have anti-inflammatory effects in the body, and researchers are just starting to explore all the possible health benefits.

A dark Chocolate a Day keeps the Doctor away

Does a dark chocolate a day keeps the doctor away?

Dark chocolate and cocoa contain several types of flavonoids, including catechin and epicatechins. Dark chocolate contains higher levels of flavanols than milk chocolate. The higher the percent cocoa, the more flavanols the chocolate contains. Many people think of dark chocolate as something their mothers used to bake with, but it has come a long way in terms of texture and flavor. Experiment with the many varieties of dark chocolate on the market to see which ones are most appealing to your tastes. Choose ones that are greater than 70 percent cocoa since a higher cocoa content contains the most flavonoids and the least amount of sugar.

Dark chocolate has been linked with lower inflammatory states in the body due to its high antioxidant activity. A 2008 study done with 5,000 people linked a square or two of dark chocolate per day with 33 percent decrease in heart disease among women and a 26 percent decrease in men. [44] The people in the study had lower levels of C-reactive protein, a marker in the blood that signals inflammation in the body.

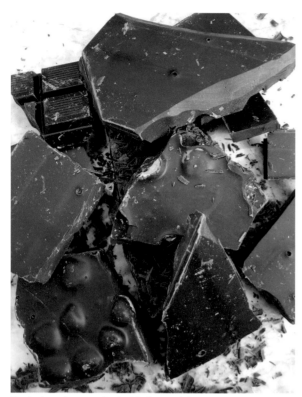
Dark chocolate: packed with flavonoids

It is recommended to eat one ounce of dark chocolate per day for health - I'd say a recommendation most of us can live with — and maybe not even a splurge, but a necessity! One of my favorite ways is having some dark chocolate shavings with berries for dessert.

And, how about a cup of tea to go with that ounce of dark chocolate?

Tea contains the polyphenol catechins and a bonus polyphenol called EGCG. Green tea contains the most EGCG of all the varieties of tea. However, all tea leaves are good sources. EGCG has been linked with a lower risk of heart disease and lower cholesterol levels. It is also associated with reduced rates of prostate, stomach and colon cancer.

Other polys worth mentioning...

Another category of non-flavonoid polyphenols have demonstrated powerful health benefits and are worth looking into. These three additional polyphenols are:

- **Resveratrol**: found in grapes and grape skins

- **Lignans**: found in the highest concentration in ground flaxseeds

- **Curcumin**: found in the spice turmeric and used to make curry

Resveratrol has shown strong anti-inflammatory effects in the body and can be helpful in prevention of atherosclerosis. **Lignans** are known as phytoestrogens inhibiting estrogen synthesis and can help prevent cancer. Flaxseed is the richest food source, but walnuts and whole grains also have lignans.

Curcumin is responsible for the yellow color in the popular Indian curry spice turmeric. Known for being an anti-inflammatory agent and antioxidant, some research shows turmeric can be helpful in preventing development of medical issues related to oxidative damage such as cancer and heart disease. It is also being studied for possible prevention or slow progression of Alzheimer's disease. Research is still in the early stages with some studies being inconclusive.

So, how can we easily pack these polyphenols into our diets?

- Grapes are a great snack anytime. Adding a piece of cheese for protein and fat achieves balance

- Top 1 tablespoon of ground flaxseed on yogurt, cottage cheese or in a salad

- Add a small amount of the spice curry or turmeric to your favorite recipes (*see Chicken Salad, Curry Scallops recipes*)

Category 3: Thiosulfonates

And lastly, thiosulfonates. A hard one to pronounce, this group of phytochemicals is important since they contain the alliums or allylic sulfides.

Allylic sulfides are a potent group of phytochemicals present in garlic, onions, shallots and leeks. Sulfur compounds have the possibility of lowering cholesterol levels, but the research is not complete as yet. They may also protect against certain carcinogens causing colon and stomach cancer.

Summary: Peel over Pill for Prevention

Without question, there are many compounds and substances in foods being discovered each day that are impossible to duplicate in vitamin supplements. Each category of phytochemicals has different protective and preventive properties, from prevention of cancer and heart disease to protection against Alzheimer's disease, MS, or fibromyalgia. Therefore, varying all the different fruits and vegetables throughout the weeks, months, and years are helpful in prevention of many types of diseases.

Taking a vitamin supplement can enhance your health in some respects, but does **not** cover your needs for phytochemicals or phytonutrients. What your mother told you may still hold true: eat a balanced diet with a variety of fruits and vegetables.

Make sure to consume a variety of color to cover all your nutrient needs, and include some dark chocolate each day for health.

Life is a blank canvas. Let the phytochemicals and flavonoids be the colors enhancing and painting your life with additional health.

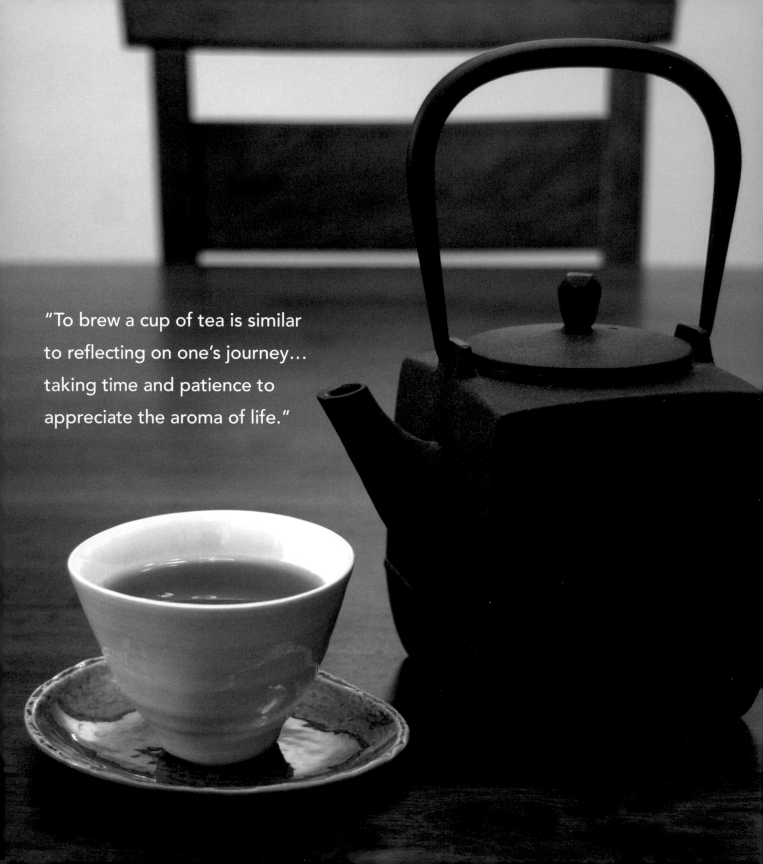

"To brew a cup of tea is similar to reflecting on one's journey... taking time and patience to appreciate the aroma of life."

Part Five

Organizing your Cooking World

Preparation for Cooking and Creating an Organized Kitchen

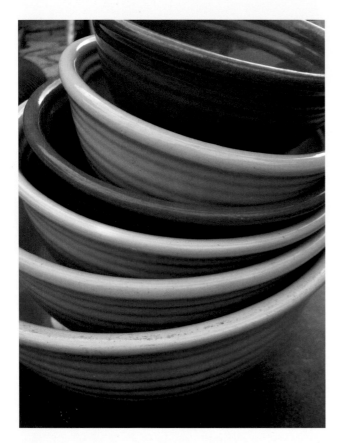

wonderful and quality appliances are great, but a small kitchen, if it's well organized, can do the same job.

Breaking it Down

Setting up for success in the kitchen is easier if you break it down into simple manageable steps.

The best way to start to organize your kitchen is to do a simple inventory. This is a big task and one you may not be able to complete at one setting. To avoid getting discouraged, view your kitchen in sections, and address one at a time.

Here are some good organizing principles to follow:

- keep what is handy

- donate what you may never use

- toss broken or unused items

- store rarely used items on higher shelves

An organized space can improve your experience creating and preparing food. Many people feel limited by the amount of space they have and that can translate into frustration with cooking. Over the years, I have organized many kitchens and prepared large meals in limited space. Granted, large open countertops are

Place like items together – i.e. pots, bakeware, utensils, and storage containers with lids. This kind of inventory allows you to evaluate your essential needs and avoid cluttering your cabinets with unnecessary items. Items you rarely use, such as holiday bakeware or cookie cutters, can also be stored on higher shelves.

Food Organization

- Make a list of the meals/menus you plan to prepare during the week. Review the ingredients on hand and make a list of necessary items for shopping. (See shopping list in this book for all of the recipes we have included.)

- Shop once or twice a week depending on your particular needs and produce availability.

- If you find yourself with extra hours on a given day, prepare additional meals. Do this by doubling the recipe (freeze the second half) or make an additional food which can be served throughout the week.

- Do the prep work for the meals in advance for easy convenience when putting the dish together. (e.g. have produce pre-washed, cut up, and measured out)

- Keep your refrigerator clean and rotate the oldest items such as produce and perishables to the front. This prevents unnecessary waste of food and saves money.

- Make sure to keep a current inventory of spices on hand. (See shopping list)

Tools in the Kitchen

Remember the set of baking pans you received at your wedding? Or perhaps the great sale you could not pass up of designer pots and pans? Or better yet, the complete culinary set that includes odd utensils you haven't used?

These additional "tools" clutter up kitchens. In addition, buying sets often decreases the quality of the product and does not stand the test of time. Quality versus quantity plays a crucial role in your culinary experience.

Stocking the kitchen shelves with middle-to-top-of-the-road cookware enhances the cooking experience. Researching the particular items you want to purchase is wise since the most expensive is not always the best quality. I would encourage experimenting with a particular brand before expanding. Then you are not locked into a cabinet full of coordinating pots that may not work for your needs.

Consider all aspects surrounding your purchase of kitchen tools, appliances, and equipment:

- cost

- longevity

- quality

- purpose and usage

The following is a list of tools which are used in all the recipes in this book:

Power/Electric
- Blender - great for soups and sauces

- Food processor – large and small/mini - chops, dices, pulses, mixes – good for pestos and sauces

Knives
There is a broad scope of different types of knives. For simplicity, let us stick to a few basic types:

- Paring (2-4 inch quality blades) – small knives used to peal, slice, or cut up smaller fruits and vegetables

- Chef's (6-12 inch quality blades) – great for chopping, cutting up vegetables, or slicing up large pieces of meats

Utensils/Equipment

- peelers - vegetables and fruit skins

- spoons – wooden and plastic

- whisks – to whip or beat eggs

- tongs – to turn and lift vegetables and meats

- spatulas – flip foods in pan or scrape pan as you cook

- grater/plainer – box with various grating sides which grate hard cheeses, fruit rinds and fresh nutmeg

- colanders – great to drain fruits, vegetables, or lettuce while preparing other items

- can opener

- meat thermometer

- timer

Measuring Utensils

2 sets each of:

- measuring cups (dry ingredients) – ¼, ⅓, ½, ⅔, ¾, 1

- glass measuring cup (liquid ingredients) – 1- ,2- and 4-cup volume

- measuring spoons – ⅛, ¼, ½, 1 teaspoons and 1 tablespoon

POTS

- **Sauce pans** – for the best heat distribution, choose stainless steel exterior and interior aluminum core with a heavy bottom and tight-fitting lids – choose small, medium, and a large stock pot.

- **Frying pans/skillet** – best sizes are 8- and 12-inch pans. Insulated handles are useful, but avoid them if you want to heat the pan in the oven.

> HINT – nonstick pans should not go from stove top to oven

Mixing Bowls – come in a variety of types – ceramic, glass, plastic, or metal. Ceramic and glass bowls have no taste or acidic interaction, or microwave heating issues.

Bakeware – comes in a variety of options, including metal, ceramic and glass

- baking dishes (9x13 is optimal size for recipes in this book)

- loaf pans

- quiche/frittata round plates/dishes

- ramekins for baking

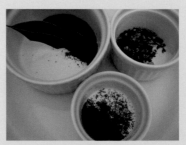

HINT – ramekins and small glass dishes are great to use during prep time to store spices, herbs, and chopped items

Clean as you Cook: Steps for Success

One key to kitchen success is adopting a clean as you go" mantra.

If you take 10-20 minutes prior to cooking for chopping, measuring, and preliminary cleanup, your culinary experience will be more enjoyable. Most of us do not have a personal sous chef to do this task. A little time spent upfront will help prevent cluttered countertops and may provide additional time to focus on cooking, presentation and perhaps engaging your family during the cooking process.

If you utilize this approach, the only items you'll have left to be washed are those used during the meal — the dinner plates, glasses, silverware, and serving dishes. Unless you are serving a large crowd, "clean as you go" can help you achieve a system whereby you do not have to face a sink full of dirty dishes later that night or the next morning.

Summary: An Organized Kitchen

No matter where you are with your current kitchen routine, just having a desire to change or make adjustments is positive and can spur movement. It is important to decide what is reasonable and to continue to build on your foundation as you progress toward better health. As time goes on, you will be able to incorporate more healthy recipes and skills toward balanced and creative eating.

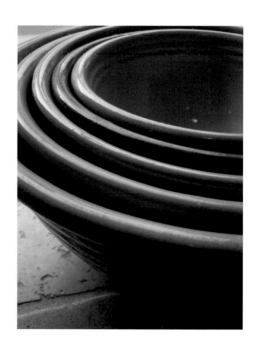

Label Reading 101

If something is designed to make our lives easier, we shouldn't feel more confused when we use it. Yet, this is how many people feel after looking at food labels. Plain and simple – food labels are not user friendly. You almost need an interpreter to figure out what information is being conveyed and how to apply it to your life. It is similar to someone who has never attempted a crossword puzzle – where do you begin?

Many things on the label are optional. For starters, we are not scientists and need only to look at key pertinent information. Percentages and the numbers at the bottom of the label are comparisons to an average male adult of a certain weight, which may or may not apply to you or others you may be shopping for. A good starting point is to read the list of ingredients on the label or side of the box. Questions to ask are:

- How many **ingredients** does the food have? If there are more than 5 or 6 ingredients, consider re-evaluating your food choice, since the more ingredients the more processed the food will be.

- Are any of the ingredients other names or components for **sugar** or starches – such as sucrose, dextrose, maltose, glucose, mannitol, sorbitol, molasses, monosaccharides, polysaccharides, maple syrup, maple sugar, date sugar, brown sugar, raw sugar, turbinado sugar, or high fructose corn syrup? If the product contains any of these, it is very likely a high-sugar product.

- Does the product contain **MSG**, or other ingredients that may contain components of MSG, such as aspartame, broth, glutamate, hydrolyzed, autolyzed yeast, monosodium glutamate, HVP, yeast extract, malted barley, rice or brown syrup? MSG is a flavor enhancer for foods, but also can increase appetite and allergic reactions in some individuals.

- How many **preservatives** or stabilizers does the product contain? Sometimes one or two are okay for a week or two of extended shelf life, but many preservatives ensure the "food" would be there next year if you came across it in your cabinet.

- Is there anything you do not recognize or can't pronounce? (a clue that it may not be a healthy food choice).

If a product contains less than five or six ingredients and does not have extras sugars or other preservatives, go ahead and check the label. Look for serving size as many manufacturers make it small (serving sizes are one of the hidden keys on a label) to make their product look healthier than it actually is. Look for "**total carbohydrates**," which will tell you how much carbohydrate/starch/sugar the product contains. 15 grams is equal to about a serving or a slice of bread. So, a product containing 45 grams of total carbohydrates is similar to consuming three slices of bread.

Trans fat is one major consideration. Unfortunately many manufacturers make the serving size so small it falls under the "do not need to report" guideline. If the serving size has less then .5 grams of trans fat, a manufacturer can state "contains no trans fat" on the label. Do not rely on what the front of the package states. If you ate several servings of a food with "no trans fat" on the label of a packaged/processed food it could add up to well over 2-3 grams of trans fat per day, which is the most dangerous type of fat.

Researchers at Harvard University, including Walter Willet, M.D., warn against consuming greater than 2 grams of trans fat per day since it can increase your risk of heart disease by 37 percent – well above any risk of consuming saturated fat. How much trans fat do processed foods contain? Check it out before purchasing. Examples include:

- a medium size order of French fries has approximately 8 grams of trans fat

- a small bag of potato chips has 5 grams

- a donut has approximately 5 grams

- a regular sized candy bar has 3 grams

If you eat even small amounts of processed foods, eating two or more grams of trans fat easily adds up.

How much **sodium** does the product contain? The average consumer eats about 6,000 mg. per day. The American Heart Association and many health organizations, including the National Academy of Sciences Institute of Medicine, recommend keeping your sodium intake below 2,300 milligrams per day. If you consume several products that contain more than 500 mg. per serving of sodium, it quickly adds up.

Summary: Label Reading

Start by looking at the list of ingredients. If the list passes the less-than-five-items litmus test, then read on to see if the product is moderate in carbohydrate, sodium, and trans fat. If it has some protein, some monounsatured fat (healthy fat) and fiber listed on the label, all the better for a balanced meal.

Otherwise, stick with fresh, unprocessed foods that do not have labels, and limit your exposure to foods in packages. The more ingredients a food contains, the longer it may take your body to process. Furthermore, if there are items you cannot pronounce or recognize on the label, it might be wise to leave it on the shelf.

Sorting through the Grocery Store Maze

The grocery store has been an interesting place for me since my childhood – it was like a toy store, but with many yummy things to eat. I remember looking at fun boxes of cereal, colorful jars of jellies and jams and begging my mother to buy "Goobers."™ The jar alone tantalized me with colorful stripes resembling a circus tent, and I loved the sticky peanut butter and grape jelly combination. I still love peanut butter, but now I eat the natural peanut butter with an apple or banana as a nutritious snack!

Food shopping has come a long way since those days. There are books dedicated to the various marketing techniques utilized by food producers, reasons processed foods cost so little, and why fresh, real food costs more. If you want to read an incredibly interesting and well-researched history book on the subject of the development of the food industry, I recommend reading Marion Nestle's book, *What to Eat*.

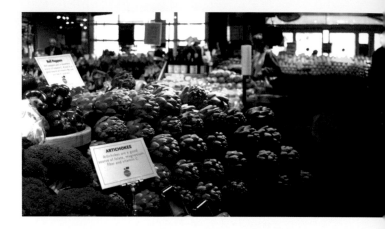

Many temptations exist in the grocery store. Especially enticing are the products on the end of the aisle that come in huge portions and are always on sale. Ninety-nine percent of these products are processed, full of trans fats, salt and sugar. It is estimated that about three quarters of the salt you consume you will never see, since it is hidden in processed foods.

Within the aisles, food manufacturers pay what is known as slotting fees, which are extra costs for their products to be placed at eye level to lure customers to their particular food. Just being conscious of these marketing techniques enables you to be an informed consumer and empowers you to be a healthy and wise shopper.

The best way to overcome the marketing ploys and end-of-aisle temptations is to be prepared with a shopping list of the items you need to prepare meals before you enter the market.

Here are some tips for success at the store:

- Make a list

- Have a plan and stay with your list

- Do not go hungry, since you will be tempted to purchase items that are not on your list (these things are often strategically placed at the end of aisles)

- If you bring children, try to feed them before you go

- Enlist your child's help with crossing things off the list, or using marketing as a teaching experience. The market is a classroom of knowledge. Teaching children about nutrients and colors in produce and where foods originated may help develop their interest in healthy eating or even science

- Stay present with what is going on, as children or teenagers will place items in the cart without your knowledge. Engage your children during checkout to help avoid the cleverly stationed candy temptations

Color Your World with Produce

So once you get yourself to the store, where to start? Many people have heard it is smart to shop on the perimeter of the grocery store. **Shopping on the periphery allows you to buy things that are fresh and wholesome, rather than processed and refined.** The produce section is a good place to start.

Most grocery stores offer organic or conventionally grown choices. Conventional foods more often are genetically modified and grown with the use of pesticides and herbicides. Organic foods are grown without the use of conventional pesticides, artificial fertilizers, human waste, or sewage sludge. Additionally, **organic foods are processed without ionizing radiation and cannot be genetically modified.**

Organic selections are usually more expensive than conventional produce. However, considering the upfront cost of not putting chemicals in your body can be a huge savings later on with increased health costs. Think of it as a financial investment with compounded interest – you can't go back and make up the deficit.

An abundance of research indicates that organic fruits and vegetables have higher levels of nutrients, including vitamin C, zinc, iron and other antioxidants. Plants grown organically develop at a normal rate and keep their nutrient levels in balance. Plants grown with conventional fertilizers develop much more quickly and have lower levels of antioxidants and nutrients. If you are not able to buy organic, buying local produce has benefits from being harvested in its prime. Since the produce does not have far to travel, it retains more nutrients, making local farmers' markets an excellent investment.

How do you decide what vegetables and fruits to buy? Most people select produce by personal preference and eat the same foods week after week. Try expanding and exploring more seasonal options. If you frequent the farmers' markets you will find what is in season and usually can buy fresh organic produce. If that option is not available to you, try to choose a variety of different fruits and vegetables. If you mix it up each week, you will rotate different nutrients for your consumption on a daily basis.

Eating fruits or vegetables with color is a good overall strategy. The more pigment the produce has, the more nutrients are present. A good slogan is: **EAT THE COLORS**. Fruits and vegetables are usually in different color categories such as purple/blue, green, orange/yellow, red and white. The color the fruit or vegetable contains identifies substances called phytochemicals that prevent disease. It is essential to **eat** the food rather than just take a pill (*see Phytochemical chapter for more information*).

Blue or purple produce will provide you with the important disease preventing phytochemicals polyphenols called *anthocyanins*. This class of produce is not

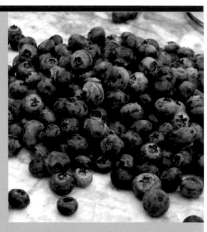

only high in antioxidants, but also known for their helpfulness in prevention of heart disease, cancer, and many inflammatory processes in the body. Some of the basic ones include:

- blackberries and blueberries
- purple grapes
- plums
- purple cabbage
- eggplant

We have heard for years that if you want to live a long life "eat green vegetables." Many people have aversions to vegetables since they can have strong flavors. If you do not have a fondness for vegetables, try having a "no thank you" serving each time a different vegetable is served. A "no thank you" serving is having a bite or two (one or two teaspoons) of something you do not particularly like each time it is served.

An easy way to try this is to have a bite of a vegetable a friend orders when you eat out. Many years ago I avoided eating avocados. I would pick them out of salads. As the research amplified the benefits of the good fats in avocado I told myself I need to train my taste buds to like them. One evening, a friend and I were out to dinner, and she ordered a salad with an overabundance of avocado slices. With my friend's permission, I took two bites of her avocado. I would have a bite or two of avocado each time I was with her, and eventually I started loving avocados.

Eating a bite or two of food that is foreign or not to your taste can change the way you feel about that food over time. Eventually your taste buds will change and you might find yourself loving certain vegetables. Like most children, I was not a vegetable lover. Even being a registered dietitian was not encouragement enough to expand my horizons. Eventually I employed the "no thank you" serving to train my taste buds to like vegetables and over time I found myself loving them!

Research has demonstrated that if you consume a food enough times you will eventually start to like it, even crave it. The same holds true for eating fast or processed food – if you consume processed food, it is what you will desire and crave. Eating healthy produce is important for your success in improving and maintaining health. To change an eating habit, you may need to find internal resolve to take the next step in realigning your food journey toward health and happiness.

Green fruits and vegetables provide the phytochemical *carotenoids* called *zeaxanthin* and *lutein*, which are helpful for eye 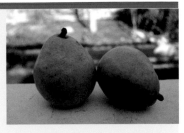 health and prevention of age-related macular degeneration. They include:

- green apples and green pears
- kiwi
- honeydew melon
- green grapes
- lettuce such as romaine, red or green leaf
- zucchini
- spinach and asparagus
- celery and cucumbers
- green beans

Nutrition Tip
If you don't like the texture or flavor of a particular fruit or vegetable, experiment by topping it with lemon, lime or orange slices to cut the strong flavor and transition your palate to like the food's taste.

An important group of vegetables that are mostly green include the **cruciferous vegetables** or brassicas. These contain many health and anti-cancer properties. Cruciferous vegetables include: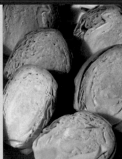

- broccoli and cauliflower
- Brussels sprouts
- bok choy
- collard greens, kale and cabbage

Orange or yellow vegetables contain the *carotenoids beta* and *alpha carotene*, which are important for their anti-cancer properties, immunity and role in cardiovascular health. Orange/yellow fruits and vegetables include: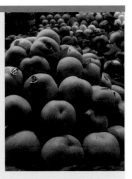

- oranges and tangerines
- pineapple
- peaches and nectarines
- grapefruit
- apricots
- lemons
- carrots
- butternut squash
- yellow or orange peppers
- sweet potatoes and yams
- pumpkin

White fruits or vegetables can contain phytochemicals known as *allylic sulfides* or *alliums*, in addition to other nutrients. Alliums protect against carcinogens causing colon or stomach cancer, in addition to lowering cholesterol levels. White fruits or vegetables include:

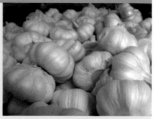

- bananas
- white nectarines or peaches
- onions, garlic and shallots
- mushrooms
- turnips and parsnips
- artichokes
- ginger

Red fruits and vegetables contain the *carotenoids lycopenes* and the *polyphenols anthocyanins* which help with cancer prevention and cardiovascular health. Red fruits and vegetables include:

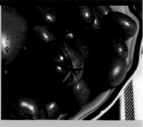

- raspberries, cranberries and strawberries
- pomegranates
- cherries
- blood red oranges
- watermelon
- red peppers
- tomatoes
- radicchio
- rhubarb
- red beets

Avocados, although technically a fruit since they have a seed, are counted as a good source of monounsaturated fat. **Avocados are a powerhouse food since they contain vitamin E, vitamin K, potassium, folic acid, vitamin B6, and fiber in addition to various carotenoids.** Avocados are recommended daily for cardiovascular and overall health.

Got Dairy?

The next stop in the grocery store is the dairy section. Many individuals and health care providers are anti-dairy and claim it is not needed after childhood. However, many studies confirm it is helpful in reducing symptoms of insulin resistance, kidney stones and osteoporosis.

Eggs are considered the highest quality protein which exists. Their amino acid profile is without comparison. At U.C. Berkeley, one of my first nutrition professors, Janet King, delivered an elaborate presentation on the quality and importance of eggs. Eggs have truly received a bad rap, and as discussed in the *Diet, Disease, and Medical Issues chapter*, are included in a healthy balanced diet. Eggs are an excellent source of protein, iron and the phytochemical lutein. Try to buy organic free-range when possible since they are free of pesticides or synthetic hormones, and are raised without antibiotics. Additionally they have higher natural omega-3 fatty acids, vitamin E and beta-carotene.

Milk exists in many different forms – whole, two percent, one percent and skim milk. For many years, people drank whole milk and are now drinking skim milk. Across the board, one percent milk has more calcium than skim, 2 percent or whole milk. It depends on the state you live in, but in California, one percent milk has the highest calcium content of all the milks (310 mg. per cup vs. 285 per cup). It also contains a good nutritional balance of carbohydrate, higher levels of protein and a little fat for some flavor and balance.

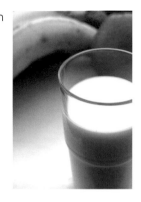

Buy organic to avoid milk produced with cows fed hormones.

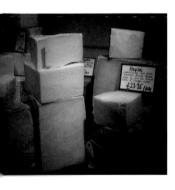

Cheese comes in many forms and has also been known as somewhat of an evil food. However, cheese is a good source of protein and calcium. If you limit your intake to two ounces per day (two nice-sized slices) it is quite reasonable in a healthy diet. Hard cheeses contain the most protein. Many imported cheese such as the Swiss cheese Emmantler is from grass-fed cows and contains omega-3 fatty acids (the anti-inflammatory fats) versus omega-6 fatty acids which are pro-inflammatory. Look for organic cheese from grass-fed cows to obtain the healthiest profile of fat. It varies depending on the time of year, since grass-feeding is not available year round in some regions.

Cottage and ricotta cheese are a good source of protein for breakfast. Low-fat cottage cheese goes well with fruit and nuts for a healthy no fuss start to the day. It is not a great source of calcium (80 mg. per half a cup) so combining it with ricotta cheese (360 mg. per half a cup) increases the calcium and palatability. Many of the recipes in this book contain ricotta cheese to add calcium and protein. It is also a great dessert with berries. For a nice

treat, locate fresh ricotta at an Italian deli, since it improves the taste in all the recipes.

Yogurt has become a manufacturer's party in terms of flavors and additives. Sometimes small containers of yogurt contain as much as 45 grams of carbohydrate or the equivalent of three slices of bread (one slice of bread contains about 15 grams of total carbohydrate). Now food manufacturers are promoting and selling yogurt as a "functional food" or a food used to prevent disease.

If you are going to eat yogurt, buy the basic, organic low fat or whole milk plain yogurt and taste several brands to decide which one you prefer. Adding fruit, nuts, seeds, and a little honey adds to the flavor and also provides your body with the good bacteria it needs (fashionably called *probiotics*). The Greek styles of yogurt available at many stores are thick and creamy and are an excellent source of calcium at 400 mg. per cup. Choosing the better-for-you yogurt is important for your health versus purchasing yogurts containing sugared fruit, sweeteners, additives and extra calories.

As stated in the *Clean Food chapter*, choose **butter** instead of margarine or sprays. Unsalted, organic regular or whipped butter is a good choice for eating or baking.

Pass the Condiments, Please

Choosing the right **oils** can be very challenging. Recommendations from the "experts" seem to change on a daily basis. Years ago, most of the population ate butter. Then, experts reported that vegetable oils were a much healthier alternative, and many people switched to corn or vegetable oils. This advice did not turn out to be true since weight, heart disease and diabetes have been rapidly increasingly. The good news is that research on which oils are healthy has become clearer during the last year. Choosing which oil to buy depends on the purpose – i.e. cooking versus using in salad dressing or baking.

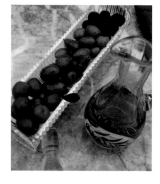

Olive oil is a monounsaturated fat that is useful in making salad dressing and marinating vegetables and meats. If you are cooking with olive oil, only use it in recipes where the smoke point is between 200 to less than 400 degrees. The best olive oil is cold-pressed, extra virgin since it contains both the good monounsaturated fat and powerful antioxidants known as *Polyphenols*. This type of olive oil means the olives are processed within 24 hours of picking, which aids in retaining a higher quality product. It is slightly cloudy due to the small particles of olive flesh in the oil. Olive oil which is clear still contains the monounsaturated fat but is devoid of the Polyphenols. "Lite" olive oil is a marketing gimmick that just refers to a milder flavor, rather than less fat and calories.

Coconut oil is a safe oil to cook with at high temperatures since it is saturated and the molecules cannot be damaged. Organic coconut oil is best since it is free of pesticides. Limit high omega-6 oils (*see Fat chapter*) such as safflower, sunflower, corn, and soybean oil.

Canola oil, although high in omega-3 fatty acids, has a high sulfur content and can quickly become rancid. It has been reported that baked goods made with canola oil can quickly develop mold. Due to the high level of rancidity, canola oil must be deodorized, and this process can increase the amount of trans fatty acids in canola oil, which negates the benefits of the omega-3 fatty acids that are present. In addition, since canola is the result of irradiated seeds from rapeseed, the oil is 80-85% GMO (*see Clean Food chapter*).

The best oils to buy are cold pressed extra virgin olive oil, organic coconut oil, and to a lesser extent flax seed oil and other nut oils such as walnut, peanut or grapeseed.

Condiments

Other condiments you may encounter or need are mayonnaise, ketchup, and sauces. Avoid barbeque and steak sauces since they can contain various additives and sugars, including high fructose corn syrup. Most mustards are healthy and a good source of flavoring in recipes, unless you need to limit your salt intake. Most ketchups contain large amounts of sugar or high fructose corn syrup. Several new brands have been developed that are unsweetened. Two tablespoons of ketchup contains 7 grams of carbohydrate or half a slice of bread. The average person uses at least 4 tablespoons of ketchup on a hamburger which is 15 carbohydrates or 1 slice of bread. Although it may take a while to enjoy a ketchup-less burger, it may be worth skipping the additional carbohydrates.

Finding a good **mayonnaise** is challenging. It is important to avoid all the "lite" low fat ones since they are full of sugar and additives. Most mayonnaises in this country are made with soybean oil, which is not only an omega-6 oil but a GMO product and needs to be minimized. It is close to impossible to find a mayonnaise made with olive oil unless you make it yourself or buy it online.

Vinegars are wonderful flavor enhancers in many recipes, adding spice and extra flavor to bland tasting foods. Choose balsamic, cider, rice, white or red vinegar, or most any one that seems interesting to add to dressings, marinades, etc. Check for additional added sugar in certain vinegars.

What about **vegetable and chicken broths**? Many brands exist on the market. It is important to buy one that is free of additives or preservatives and lower in sodium. For example, many popular brands contain MSG, and/or list one of the 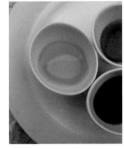 ingredients as "broth" which can contain forms of MSG. Therefore, it is important to choose a brand that does not contain MSG or the word broth in the label (*see Clean Food chapter*). Choose organic, low sodium, prepared with vegetables, herbs or spices for the best flavored broth. A good option is to make your own.

Spice It Up

Salt is the universal spice to improve flavor. There are also rich sources of ground and fresh spices. Adding spices greatly enhances any dish. We have carefully chosen particular spices for the recipes in this book. How do we differentiate the types of salt? Salt can be obtained from two sources: rock formations that are mined, or from the ocean by evaporating the water, leaving the salt.

What is the healthiest salt?

Table salt exists in iodized and non-iodized form. It is made from rock salt, and goes through a refining process removing naturally occurring minerals and adds chemicals to prevent clumping. This process results in the ground and refined forms of salt sold in the store. Morton Salt Company began adding iodine to salt in 1924 to decrease the chance of goiters, which have been greatly reduced.

Sea salt is made from evaporating ocean water and is available in both fine and course grains. It may contain some trace minerals such as iodine,

magnesium and potassium. Some varieties available from India are pink or brown. There are also those from France that are usually gray in color and have fancy names such as *Fleur de Sel*.

Kosher salt is made from sea water or salt mines and is used for curing meats and kosher foods. It contains no additives or added iodine and is considered better than table salt from a nutritional standpoint since it contains less sodium. Kosher salt is frequently used by chefs because of the course texture and ease with picking up and sprinkling it on foods.

Rock salt is one you may remember from making home-made ice-cream where ice and rock salt are combined in a hand cranking ice-cream maker. It is sold as large crystals.

Organic salt is similar to table salt, but contains no additives or chemicals.

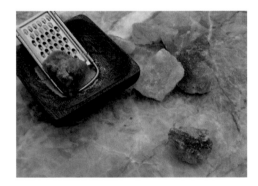

If you are using salt, kosher or sea salt are better choices due to the natural minerals and slightly less sodium content. Use sparingly and use fresh or ground spices to flavor foods and observe how good food can taste with less added salt.

Meat, Poultry and Fish

The next section of the store is the meat, poultry and fish section. Many choices exist: grass-fed vs. corn-fed meat, farmed vs. wild fish, etc. Grass-fed meat tastes different but is far healthier than corn-fed meat, although again more expensive. Grass-fed meat also contains more omega-3 fatty acids versus the omega-6 fatty acids corn-fed meat contains. It also contains higher levels of CLA's (conjugated linoleic acids) which have been linked to lowering inflammation, diabetes, cancer, and increasing immunity.

- **Certified organic** meats or poultry are free of pesticides, hormones or antibiotic residues, giving assurance that the cattle were raised in a more humane manner. The feed is entirely vegetarian and the animals have access to pastureland, exercise and sunlight. The USDA regulates the animals throughout their lives, including feed sources and medication.

- **Certified** humane means the meat or poultry is free of antibiotics, growth hormones, and is regulated by the USDA, but does not have the other restrictions of certified organic.

- **Natural** just means that the meat or poultry was processed without additives or preservatives. These labels are not regulated by the USDA, so you can never be sure what you are truly buying!

Most of the beef in this country is from corn/grain-fed animals. Corn/grain-fed beef comes from an animal fed a combination of grass and grains along with vitamin and mineral supplements. Grass-fed or grass-finished meat comes from animals eating only a diet of grass and who remain on a pasture their entire lives. Most grass-fed beef is imported from Australia and New Zealand where grass is in greater abundance and grows year round. However, more grass-fed meat is becoming available in the U.S. due to demand and the health benefits it provides.

Minding your Meats

If you stick to lean sources of meat (filet, loin, and round) vs. a fatty steak or prime rib, you are consuming far less fat and calories.

- One 4-ounce piece of prime rib contains 39 grams of total fat

- One 4-ounce piece of filet mignon contains 6 grams of total fat

- Some leaner cuts of meat include: eye of the round, top sirloin, 7-15 percent ground beef, round steak, filet mignon and rump roast

Look for pink or red pigments in the meat. If the meat is dark brown, green or black, avoid these cuts as they are old and spoiled. Find a reliable butcher shop or supermarket selling fresh meat, as many butchers pull and repackage meat to present as fresh, when in fact it is old or close to the expiration date. Another tip is to buy the meat on the bottom (vs. the top of the case) since the top meat is exposed to the

> **Helpful Hint:**
> Take time to get to know your local butcher. Whether in a large or small city, butchers are trained and knowledgeable in cuts of meats. Taking the time to invest in a relationship with a butcher will pay off in the long run since they can order and cut/trim meat for you, rather than just buying what is available in the standard packages.

most air and can spoil more rapidly. Meat provides protein, iron, B-vitamins such as B-6 and B-12, zinc, selenium and a host of other nutrients essential to health.

Poultry

White meat chicken and turkey such as the breasts, and skinless dark meat are the healthiest forms of poultry. Poultry is a good source of protein, vitamin B-6, niacin (vitamin B-3) and selenium. The cuts should not have a pungent smell when purchased and need to be opaque and spot-free. Look for breasts that have a solid and plump shape, and make sure to check the expiration date.

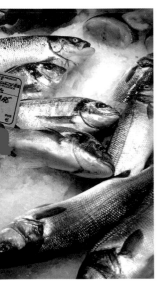

: high in omega-3 fatty acids

Fish

Fish is a loaded topic in this country requiring consumers to invest in research to actually discover what is best to purchase. Many fish are grown in mercury-rich waters and are unhealthy to consume. Wild fish vs. farmed fish have far less mercury and provide the omega-3 fatty acids that are essential to health. Some farmed fish, including farmed salmon, can contain PCBs (polychlorinated biphenyls) which are neurotoxic, hormone-disrupting chemicals that were banned in the U.S. in 1977.

It is recommended to avoid the highest mercury containing fish such as king mackerel, swordfish, Atlantic halibut, pike, shark, sea bass, and tilefish (also known as golden snapper), and canned white albacore tuna.

At the time of this writing, healthy or low mercury fish include: Arctic char, crawfish, Pacific flounder, herring, king crab, sandabs, scallops, Pacific sole,

tilapia, wild Alaska and Pacific salmon, Pacific halibut, striped bass and sturgeon. Check fish safety Web sites before purchasing fresh fish since the recommendations change. An excellent Web site to check for fish safety and mercury levels is: http://www.mbayaq.org/cr/seafoodwatch.asp.

Canned tuna is extremely over processed in this country, which makes it devoid of omega-3 fatty acids. However, it is a good source of protein. White tuna in water contains higher levels of mercury, and it is recommended that you purchase light tuna in water since it contains about a third less mercury than white. Oil-packed tuna is usually packed in an omega-6 fat, so it is best to purchase tuna packed in water.

Go Nuts for Nuts

Depending on your grocery store, the nuts and seeds will be in different locations. Stick to raw or dry roasted unsalted nuts. Raw nuts have the most beneficial fats in them, and dry roasted have approximately 10% less due to the roasting process.

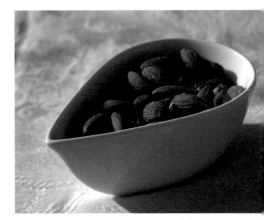

Almonds: high in monounsaturated fat

Nuts are a favorite snack food since they are easy, portable and satiating. Many people think of them as fattening. Nuts contain the good monounsaturated fat. A one ounce portion of nuts is about 180 calories and a one-ounce portion of pretzels is about 110 calories. The nuts are nutritious, are only 70 calories more and better for your health.

Almonds, walnuts, cashews, pecans, macadamias, pine nuts, and pistachios are all good choices. Make your own nut mix. There is a healthy nut mix in the Recipes section that is easy to make and tasty enough on its own or on yogurt or other foods. Sunflower and pumpkin seeds are also good choices and are a nice alternative to nuts.

Nut butters such as peanut, almond and cashew butter are a wonderful snack food and go well with apples, carrots, bananas and celery. Some of the old-fashioned peanut butters are a turn off since the oil does not mix well with the nuts. However, some great new brands are available, and if you put a knife in them and stir well, they do not separate. A client recently referred to cashew butter as dessert on a stick. Try different ones and you'll see how the rich, nutty taste can be a nice substitute for dessert and is very filling.

Against the Grains and Starches

Grains can be the more boring parts of the grocery store. Most of this book is aimed at consuming nutrient-dense foods. Pasta or potatoes contain large amounts of carbohydrate and are high glycemic index or filler foods. If you exercise several hours a day and need extra calories to keep weight on, these foods are fine. However, if you need to maximize nutrients and want to lose weight, concentrate on adequate protein intake, fruits, vegetables and salads with some whole grains to round out your meal.

Brown or wild rice and quinoa contain high levels of fiber. Consuming a moderate amount of these foods is acceptable since they are truly whole grains. Beans also contain high levels of fiber and nutrients. Buckwheat is actually not a grain but rather a fruit, making the name deceptive. It is great for those with wheat sensitivity, since it is gluten free.

Having a small serving of yams or sweet potatoes is a good choice since they contain vitamin C, B6, potassium, fiber and phytochemicals. They are filling, and readily satisfy a sweet craving for many people.

The bread section can be quite daunting. It is difficult to find a healthy bread. Bread is not a true whole grain since it is a man-made food. Whole grain wheat bread contains three parts:

- The outer part or the bran

- The inner part or the germ

- The part in between known as the endosperm

Whole wheat bread has all three parts, and white bread contains only the endosperm, taking out two parts that contain both fiber and nutrients. Look for breads with the first ingredient listed as "whole wheat or whole wheat flour." If it says "wheat flour" it is processed. Choose breads that only have a few ingredients. If you spend time in the bread section, you may observe the list of ingredients in many types of bread is quite extensive with many containing preservatives, additives and sweeteners. It may be possible to find only one brand of bread meeting your healthy criteria.

Whole wheat bread contains many more nutrients that white bread such as fiber, folic acid, vitamins B6 and E, zinc and chromium. Most white breads are enriched but they still do not contain the nutritional profile of whole wheat bread. If you choose to include bread in your diet, choose a whole wheat type and remember that it a carbohydrate source. If you are insulin resistant, it is important to limit the amount of bread ingested or remove it from your menu entirely.

Beverages

What about beverages? For many years, most people drank coffee, tea, water, milk and rarely had sodas or punch for parties or special occasions. If you spend even 5 minutes in the beverage aisle, every possible combination of soft drink, specialty coffee drink, and vitamin and flavored waters exist. Most of us do not realize that these foods have calories in them, and drinkable calories do not register in the body as satiating like solid calories in food. Food provides the nutrients we need, and obtaining it from beverages does not make sense unless you have a medical problem that hinders you from eating.

Choose water, milk, iced or hot tea without sweeteners, or natural flavored sparkling or regular water as part of a clean diet. Limit juices, since it is far healthier to eat the whole fruit which contains the pulp and fiber. **The amount of carbohydrate in a cup of juice is equal to the amount of carbohydrate or sugar in a regular soda.** Although you are also receiving vitamins in the juice, the calories add up quickly and can be deceptive. Adding a small amount of fresh lemon, lime or orange squeezed from the fruit can spruce up the taste of plain or sparkling water. *See Beverages and Fluid Intake chapter.*

Deli and Bakery

The deli counter can be friend or foe. There can be a nice selection of hard cheeses, which you can order sliced by the pound. Choose nitrate-free organic, low salt deli meats when available. If the store has salads or other prepared foods, look for protein or vegetable dishes that are made without sugars or sweeteners, corn or omega-6 rich oils, MSG or other added flavorings.

Don't always follow your nose!

The pleasant smells wafting from the bakery counter are more than tantalizing, and it is not reasonable to avoid all desserts in general. Home made is better – you can choose the ingredients and make fresh, quality desserts. Most bakeries use margarine and a host of additives in their cakes, desserts and cookies. If you read the labels, a frosted cookie can contain 25 ingredients, including margarine, many additives, preservatives and food dyes. The longer the list, the longer it takes your body to process this type of food. Remember the ingredient list in the grocery store cake in the *Fat chapter*?

Are We There Yet?

In summary, choose whole, unprocessed foods. In an optimal world, we could all buy grass-fed meat, wild fish, organic fruits and vegetables from local farmer's markets, and whole foods in their natural state. Obtaining these foods can be challenging – both in availability and affordability. Feed yourself or your family all the fresh food you can afford, and soon you will be enjoying the pleasure of unprocessed food.

Useful Information

Dry Spices

Allspice
Basil
Black pepper
Chili powder
Cinnamon
Cumin
Curry powder
Dill
Garlic powder
Ginger
Herb de Provence
Italian spice
Nutmeg
Oregano
Red pepper flakes
Sage*
Sea or Kosher salt
*only in Pork with apples/
carrots

Fresh Herbs

Fennel bulb & fronds
Garlic
Ginger
Lemon juice
Onions
Italian parsley
Shallots
Basil
Rosemary*
*used in Rosemary Lemon
Lamb

Condiments

Butter
Coconut oil
Dijon mustard
Mustard
Kalamata olives
Low-salt chicken broth
Low-salt vegetable
  broth
Olive oil

Vinegars

Apple cider vinegar
Balsamic vinegar
Red wine vinegar
White balsamic vinegar

Canned Goods

Canned pumpkin
Garbanzo beans
Low-salt diced
  tomatoes
Low-salt tomato puree
Red kidney beans
Tomato paste

Nuts/Seeds

Almonds
Cashews
Ground flax seeds
Macadamia nuts
Pecans
Pine nuts
Pumpkin seeds
Sunflower seeds

Vegetables

Asparagus
Bean sprouts
Broccoli
Brussels sprouts
Butternut squash
Carrots
Cauliflower
Celery
Cucumber
Eggplant
Lettuce
Mushrooms
Peppers-orange/
  red
Tomatoes
Yams
Yellow squash
Zucchini

Fruits

Apples
Avocados
Berries
Grapefruit
Lemon
Nectarines
Oranges
Peaches

Proteins

Beef filet
Chicken breast
Eggs
Ground beef
Ground turkey
Lamb chops
New York strip
Pork chops
Pork tenderloin
Scallops
Tilapia
Turkey tenderloins
Wild salmon

Dairy

1% milk
Cream
Feta cheese
Monterey Jack
Mozzarella cheese
Parmesan cheese
Plain yogurt
Provolone cheese
Ricotta cheese
Sour cream

Grains

Buckwheat flour
Steel-cut oats
Whole wheat flour

Baking Items

Espresso powder
Honey
Semi-sweet
  chocolate chips
100% cane sugar
Vanilla extract

Miscellaneous

Sun-dried tomatoes
  in oil
Unsweetened
  coconut

Holiday

Dried dates
Healthy wheat bread
Italian sausage
Marjoram, fresh
Persimmons
Sage, fresh
Thyme, fresh

NOT TO SHOP

You may find it helpful to bring the following list to the grocery store. Look carefully at the labels to see if any of these ingredients are contained in products you're considering. Some of them are hidden names for MSG, sugars or sweeteners or hidden genetically modified sources.

Acesulfame-K	Gelatin	Monosodium glutamate (MSG)
Aspartame	Glutamate	Potassium bromate
Autolyzed yeast	Glutamic acid	Propyl gallate
BHT, BHA	Glycerin, glycerol, glycerol monooleate	Rice or brown syrup
Broth	Glycine	Saccharin
Canola oil	High fructose corn syrup (HFCS)	Sorbitol
Casein or Caseinate	Hydrogenated fat	Soy – flour, lecithin, protein, isolate, isoflavone
Corn - flour, meal, oil, starch, gluten, and syrup	Hydrolyzed	Soybean oil
Cottonseed oil	Hydrolyzed vegetable protein (HVP)	Sucralose
Crystalline fructose	Malted Barley	Vegetable - oil and protein
Dextrose, glucose, dextrin, sucrose, maltose	Maltitol, Mannitol	Xanthan gum
Flavorings (including "natural" flavorings), emulsifiers, stabilizers	Modified food starch	Yeast extract
Food colorings (Blue, Red Green, Yellow)	Monosaccharides Polysaccharides	

More information about the items on this list can be found at www.mercola.com and www.centerforfoodsafety.org

Quick Guide to Cooking Temperatures

Beef – is best cooked to a minimal temperature of 145° F, which is considered medium rare to medium. **Buy a meat thermometer if you don't have one.**

Ground Beef – needs to cook to a minimal temperature of 160° F. The Centers for Disease Control and Prevention (CDC) advises against eating pink, undercooked ground meat as it increases your risk for food-borne illness.

Lamb – best cooked to a minimum temperature of 140° F for medium rare.

Poultry – best cooked to minimum temperature of 165° F. Your personal preference may indicate a higher temperature.

Seafood – cook most fish until 145° F or opaque.

Eggs – are best cooked until yolks and whites are firm. It is unadvisable to use recipes which call for raw or partially cooked eggs.

USDA Recommended Safe Minimum Internal Temperatures

Steaks and roasts	145 °F
Fish	145 °F
Pork	160 °F
Ground beef	160 °F
Egg dishes	160 °F
Chicken breasts	165 °F
Whole poultry	165 °F

These lists can be downloaded for use in shopping at www.susandopart.com

Cooking Desire

Find the Chef in You!

A message from Jeffrey

My earliest memory in the kitchen was when I was about three years old. I recall standing on top of a yellow stool with my grandma making butterfly pancakes. She encouraged me at an early age to explore and be creative with food, which spurred my lifelong desire to experiment in the kitchen and create interesting food.

If you compare your living space to the body as a whole, the kitchen is like the heart, pumping nutrients throughout the house and feeding those who live there. Perhaps this is why people like to gather in the kitchen during social occasions. It represents the heart of togetherness.

Over the years, I have been blessed to learn cooking techniques and culinary heritage from wonderful people. After Susan and I were married, I was introduced to Italian cooking by her aunts, Lydia and Tooter. I've been privileged to learn their family secrets to create wonderful tasting sauces and flavorful dishes. With no formal outside training, my own culinary experience has been enriched by the kindness and help of others – proof a person can create healthy, clean food without being a chef.

Purpose of our recipes

The recipes that follow are designed for convenience, simplicity and health. We felt it was important to develop them from an organic concept and maintain this integrity throughout each recipe.

Our goal was to create recipes with home-cooked flavor that will work within economic and time constraints. We wanted you, the cook, to explore

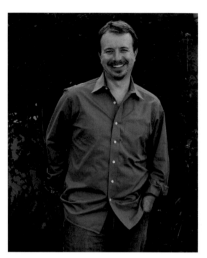

your culinary skills and satisfy your sense of taste by being able to add variations to the base menus. By either increasing or decreasing the spices and exploring healthy variations, our hope is to increase your confidence level in the kitchen.

Food preparation can be an enjoyable experience, not just a required chore. We want to inspire and empower you to create healthy meals for yourself and your family. By being equipped and prepared, you can take pleasure in healthy eating and restore balance in your life. Helping you on that journey is our purpose in writing this book.

We have provided a shopping list for your convenience. If you have all the ingredients on the list on hand, you will be able to make any recipe in this book. A "Not to Shop" list is also provided for ingredients to limit or avoid when shopping.

Our goal is to help you take pleasure in healthy, restorative eating.

Bon appétit!

Part Six

Recipes For Health and Good Eating

French New York Strip

Servings: 4 4-ounce
Prep Time: 5 mins
Cook Time: 12-18 mins

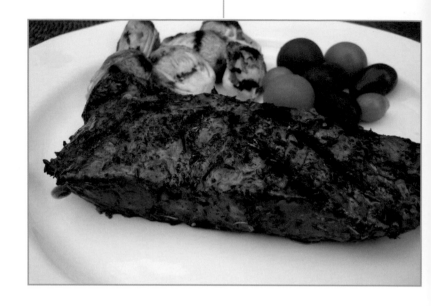

Ingredients:

1¼ pounds **of grass-fed New York strip**

½ teaspoon **Herbs de Provence**

¼ teaspoon **garlic powder**

⅛ teaspoon **red pepper flakes**

1½ tablespoons **olive oil, divided**

Preparation:

Preheat oven to 400 degrees.

Mix together spices to make a dry rub and set aside. Coat meat with ½ tablespoon of olive oil, and then cover meat with the dry rub mixture.

Sear meat in an ovenproof skillet with remaining tablespoon of olive oil over medium heat for approximately 3-4 minutes. Flip meat over, and cook for an additional 1-2 minutes. Place in oven and finish cooking until desired doneness is achieved, approximately 6-8 minutes for steaks cooked to medium doneness.

Variation: Can be cooked on grill.

Recipe and Nutrition Tip:
Bring meat to room temperature approximately 10-20 minutes before cooking, which helps with even cooking. Grass-fed meat contains higher amounts of omega-3 fatty acids than corn or grain-fed meat.

Nutrition Facts	Per Serving
Calories	202
Protein	25 grams
Total Carbohydrates	0 grams
Total Fat	10 grams
Fiber	0 grams
Sodium	67 mg.

Orange Flax Filet Mignon

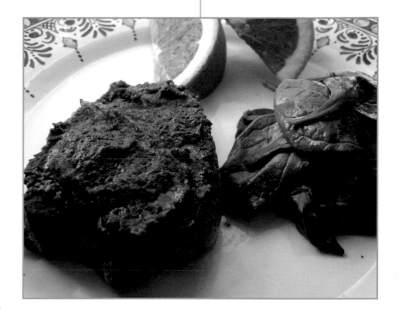

Ingredients:

4 **filet mignons (about 4 ounces each)**

2 tablespoons **ground flaxseed**

1 tablespoon **Dijon mustard**

½ teaspoon **finely-grated, fresh orange zest**

Salt and pepper to taste

1 tablespoon **olive oil**

Preparation:

Preheat oven to 500 degrees.

Make a paste of ground flaxseed, mustard, orange zest, and salt and pepper to taste.

Heat oil in an oven-proof skillet over medium heat until shimmering. Sear the steaks for 3-5 minutes until brown on one side. Remove from heat, and turn steaks over.

Spread the rub on the seared side and put the skillet in the oven for 6-8 minutes until desired doneness.

Total cooking time: 8-10 minutes for medium rare steaks.

Nutrition Tip:
An easy way to increase ground flaxseed in your diet, high in omega-3 fatty acids.

Nutrition Facts	Per Serving
Calories	176
Protein	23 grams
Total Carbohydrates	2 grams
Total Fat	9 grams
Fiber	1 gram
Sodium	145 mg.

Meatballs

Servings: 15 meatballs
Prep Time: 20 mins
Cook Time: 15-20 mins

Ingredients:

1½ tablespoons **olive oil, divided**

½ **large, sweet yellow onion, diced**

4 **cloves garlic, minced**

1 pound **85% lean ground beef**

2 **large eggs**

2 tablespoons **ground flaxseed**

2 tablespoons **parmesan cheese**

½ cup **chopped fresh Italian parsley**

1 teaspoon **ground oregano**

Salt and pepper to taste

Recipe and Nutrition Tip:
The ground flaxseed replaces the bread crumbs in traditional recipes and gives the meatballs their moistness as well as increasing omega-3 fatty acids.

For healthier cooking, place meatballs on oven-proof rack on cookie sheet and bake to allow extra fat to drip off.

Nutrition Facts	Per Meatball
Calories	111
Protein	10 grams
Total Carbohydrates	1.3 grams
Total Fat	7 grams
Fiber	.5 grams
Sodium	48 mg.

Preparation:

In a large skillet, sauté 1 tablespoon of olive oil and onions over medium heat for 4-5 minutes. Add garlic and continue to cook until tender and soft. Remove from heat and place in large mixing bowl. Let cool for 5 minutes.

In the same bowl, thoroughly mix meat, eggs, ground flaxseed, cheese, parsley and dry spices. (Best to mix with hands.)

Form round balls approximately 1 inch diameter, continually dipping fingers in a glass of cold water to prevent sticking. Place the uncooked meat balls on a plate until completed.

Pan fry method:
In batches, add the remaining oil and sauté while carefully turning meatballs to make sure they are fully cooked. Then add to sauce to complete cooking if desired.

Oven method:
Heat oven to 400 degrees and place meatballs on a cookie sheet for 20-25 minutes. Turn meatballs over halfway through for even cooking.

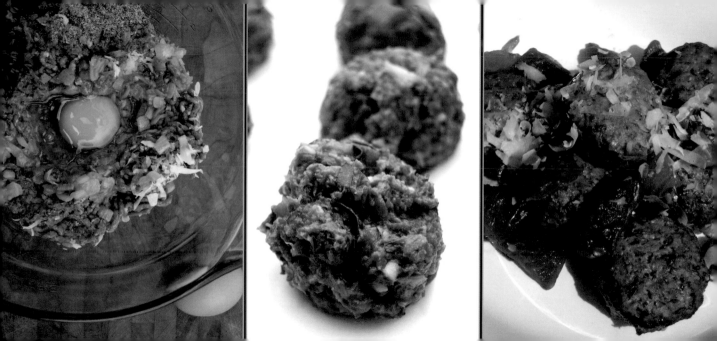

Simple Burgers

Servings: 4
Prep Time: 5 mins
Cook Time: 7-12 mins

Ingredients:

1 pound of 85% lean ground beef

1-2 tablespoons Italian spice

1-2 tablespoons grated parmesan cheese

1 large egg

Salt and pepper to taste

½ tablespoon olive oil

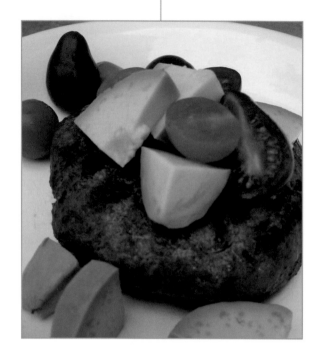

Preparation:

Mix first five ingredients together and form into 4 patties. Sauté patties in pan over medium heat in the olive oil until desired doneness, flipping patties halfway through cooking.

Variation: Can be made on grill, or substitute ground turkey or chicken.

Recipe Tip:
Dress up these burgers with avocado, tomato slices, or melted cheese. Good for an easy meal anytime.

Nutrition Facts	Per Serving
Calories	338
Protein	33 grams
Total Carbohydrates	1 gram
Total Fat	21 grams
Fiber	.5 grams
Sodium	158 mg.

Spicy Meat Chili

Servings: 12 one-cup servings
Prep Time: 10-15 mins
Cook Time: 60-90 mins

Ingredients:

6 garlic cloves, peeled and chopped

1½ medium yellow onions, chopped

1 medium red bell pepper, seeded and diced

2 tablespoons olive oil

2 tablespoons chili powder

1 tablespoon cumin

1 teaspoon red pepper flakes

1 teaspoon oregano

2 pounds 85% lean ground beef

One 28-ounce can low salt tomato puree

One 28-ounce can low salt diced tomatoes

One 15-ounce can dark red kidney beans, drained

Salt and pepper to taste

Lime or lemon wedges

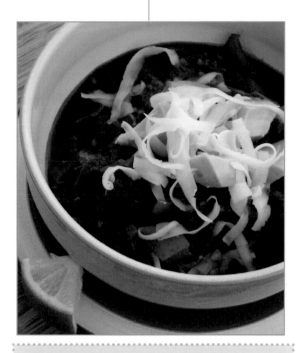

Preparation:

In a Dutch oven or a large stockpot, sauté garlic, onions, red pepper and all the dry spices in olive oil. Stir continually over medium heat until vegetables are soft, approximately 8 to 10 minutes. Increase heat to high and mix in ground beef. Continue cooking until beef is completely cooked or no longer pink. Add tomato puree, tomatoes, and kidney beans. Bring to a boil.

Reduce heat, simmer and cover stirring occasionally for 45 minutes. Remove cover and continue to cook for an additional 30 minutes. If chili becomes too thick or sticks to the pan, add water in half cup increments. Enjoy with lime or lemon wedges.

Recipe Tip:
One of the keys to creating a successful chili is balancing the spicy, hot, and sweet flavors. Letting the flavors blend over a period of time makes this process more successful. This chili has a tomato base with a heavy focus on protein and spices to please the palate. Adjust the spices to your liking. This recipe makes a lot to allow for leftovers or for freezing half and enjoying later.

Nutrition Facts	Per Serving
Calories	302
Protein	24 grams
Total Carbohydrates	17 grams
Total Fat	15 grams
Fiber	5 grams
Sodium	183 mg.

Chicken with Feta and Tomato Sauce

Servings: 4
Prep Time: 15 mins
Cook Time: 30 mins

Ingredients:

4 boneless chicken breast halves

(about 4 ounces each or a total of one pound)

1 tablespoon olive oil, divided

2 large shallots, sliced

½ tablespoon dried oregano

One 15-ounce can tomato puree

1 cup low-salt chicken broth

¾ cup feta cheese

⅓ cup chopped black olives (Kalamata preferred)

Salt and pepper to taste

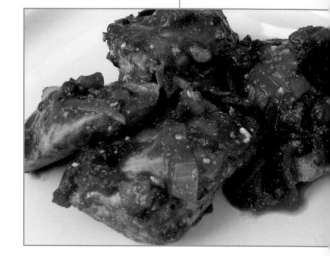

Preparation:

Rub chicken with ½ tablespoon of olive oil and season with salt and pepper if desired.

Heat ½ tablespoon of oil in large heavy skillet over medium heat. Sauté shallots until tender, approximately 5 minutes. Add chicken to skillet and sauté until golden brown. Turn chicken over and cook an additional 2-3 minutes, or 4-5 minutes total time.

Add oregano, tomato puree and broth; cover and bring to a boil. Reduce heat to medium-low. Simmer until chicken is just cooked through, about 10-12 minutes or until juices run clear. Remove chicken from pan.

Increase heat to thicken sauce adding in cheese and olives, cooking for about 5-7 minutes.

Return chicken to sauce and simmer for another 5 minutes until heated through.

Recipe Tip:
This Greek-inspired dish is a hearty pleaser and makes great leftovers. Double the recipe for a second night or freeze for a rainy day. Great for transporting to a party – just prepare and reheat in microwave or oven.

Nutrition Facts	Per Serving
Calories	318
Protein	33 grams
Total Carbohydrates	15 grams
Total Fat	14 grams
Fiber	2.5 grams
Sodium	700 mg.

High-Protein Lasagna

Servings: 8
Prep Time: 60-90 mins
Cook Time: 45 mins

Ingredients:

1½ **pounds of shredded chicken breast**

1 **medium eggplant, about 2 pounds**

1 **medium red bell pepper, cored and seeded**

1 **medium yellow red pepper, cored and seeded**

2 **medium zucchini**

2 **medium crookneck yellow squash**

2 tablespoons **olive oil**

3 cups **part-skim mozzarella cheese**

2 cups **part-skim ricotta cheese**

4 cups **easy tomato sauce (see recipe)**

Recipe and Nutrition Tip:
A great recipe to incorporate the tastes of different types of vegetables. Makes a large amount and freezes well.

Nutrition Facts	Per Serving
Calories	315
Protein	22 grams
Total Carbohydrates	14 grams
Total Fat	19 grams
Fiber	3.5 grams
Sodium	402 mg.

Preparation:

Boil boneless skinless chicken breasts in a stockpot of water with a pinch of salt. The longer you cook the chicken the more tender it becomes. Cook on high for approximately 1-1.5 hours. Rinse under cold water and shred apart with a fork.

Cut ends of eggplant off, and a slice into ¼ inch medallions. Slice squashes into ¼ inch medallions. Thinly slice peppers. Sauté or roast all vegetables in olive oil until soft.

Mix together mozzarella and ricotta cheeses in a separate bowl.

In a large glass pan (approximately 9.5 x 13.5), place 3 layers of ingredients. First, put about 2 cups of sauce on the bottom of the pan. Then layer one third eggplant, squashes, peppers (vegetables), shredded chicken, and cheese mixture. For the second layer use one cup of sauce, another third of the vegetables, chicken, and cheese mixture. Top with remaining chicken, vegetables, sauce and cheese mixture.

Bake at 350 degrees for 30-45 minutes. Let stand 15 minutes before serving.

Variation: In place of shredded chicken, you can use baked chicken, cooked ground beef or poultry, or exclude meat for a vegetarian dish.

Lemon Chicken

Servings: 4
Prep Time: 15 mins
Cook Time: 20 mins

Ingredients:

1 pound chicken breasts, pounded to ¼ inch thickness

2 tablespoons whole wheat flour

2 tablespoons olive oil, divided

¼ cup chopped yellow onions

1 large clove garlic, minced

1 medium lemon, thinly sliced

Juice of 1 medium lemon

1 cup low sodium chicken broth

1½ tablespoons butter

2 tablespoons Italian parsley

Salt and pepper to taste

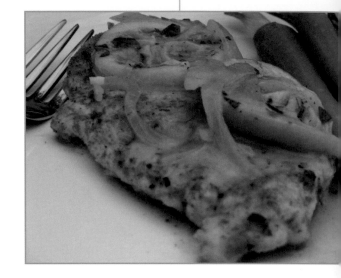

Preparation:

Preheat oven to 200 degrees, with a heat-proof plate on rack.

Lightly salt and pepper chicken to taste. Lightly dredge the pounded chicken breasts in flour. Heat 1 tablespoon of olive oil and sauté ½ the chicken breasts until golden brown, approximately 2-3 minutes on each side. Once chicken is cooked, put on plate in the oven to keep chicken warm. Repeat with the other tablespoon of olive oil and remaining chicken.

Using the same pan, sauté the onions over medium heat adding the garlic after about 30 seconds and sauté for an additional 45 seconds. Add the lemon slices and chicken broth, and increase the temperature slightly stirring often until the liquid is reduced by half. Add the lemon juice and lower heat to simmer. Add in butter and stir to thicken sauce. Add parsley at the end and pour mixture over the chicken.

Recipe and Nutrition Tip:
A lemon lover's delight full of tangy flavors. Even more flavorful if the lemons are thinly sliced and sautéed a bit longer. If you have a lemon tree or know someone who does, using homegrown lemons brings more richness to this dish.

Nutrition Facts	Per Serving
Calories	294
Protein	35 grams
Total Carbohydrates	7 grams
Total Fat	13 grams
Fiber	1.3 grams
Sodium	163 mg.

Tangy Tomato Basil Chicken

Servings: 4
Prep Time: 10 mins
Cook Time: 20 mins

Ingredients:

1 pound **chicken breasts (4 4-ounces breasts, boneless and skinless)**

½ teaspoon **ground pepper**

1 tablespoon **olive oil**

½ **sweet yellow onion, sliced**

2 **garlic cloves, minced**

1 **14.5-ounce can low-salt diced tomatoes**

3 tablespoons **white balsamic or rice wine vinegar**

¼ cup **thinly sliced fresh basil leaves, divided**

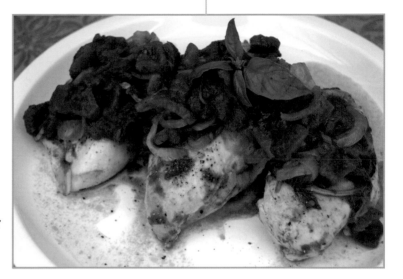

Preparation:

Pepper each side of chicken. Heat olive oil in a large skillet over medium heat. Sauté onions and garlic until translucent and tender, 6-7 minutes. Add chicken breasts and cook an additional 4 minutes on each side or until golden brown.

Add the diced tomatoes and vinegar. Reduce heat and add basil. Continue cooking until juices run clear, approximately 4-5 minutes.

Top with fresh basil, if desired.

Recipe Tip:
Surprisingly simple with a bountiful bouquet of flavors.

Nutrition Facts	Per Serving
Calories	222
Protein	34 grams
Total Carbohydrates	7 grams
Total Fat	5 grams
Fiber	1 gram
Sodium	97 mg.

Turkey Tenderloins with Pesto and Provolone

Servings: 4
Prep Time: 15 mins (with pesto)
Cook Time: 10 mins

Ingredients:

1 pound turkey tenderloins, pounded, or turkey breast cutlets

1 teaspoon olive oil

4 tablespoons sun-dried tomato pesto (see recipe)

4 slices of provolone, approximately 1 ounce each

Recipe and Nutrition Tip:
A quick dinner that can be made in less than 10 minutes if you have turkey or chicken in the house. The pesto can be made ahead of time and keeps for 2-3 weeks in the refrigerator.

Nutrition Facts	Per Serving
Calories	264
Protein	36 grams
Total Carbohydrates	2 grams
Total Fat	13 grams
Fiber	.6 grams
Sodium	330 mg.

Preparation:

Preheat oven to 375 degrees.

If using tenderloins, pound to a ¼ inch thickness. Sauté turkey in olive oil over medium heat, cooking about 1-3 minutes per side, or until juices run clear. While sautéing the second side, put 1 tablespoon of pesto on tenderloin and cover with 1 slice of cheese.

Transfer to an oven safe plate and put in oven for a minute or two to melt cheese. Serve immediately.

Variation: Cover pan to melt cheese instead of using oven.

134 | Recipes: Poultry

Victoria Turkey Burgers

Servings: 4
Prep Time: 30 mins
(including refrigeration)
Cook Time: 12-15 mins

Ingredients:

2 teaspoons **olive oil, divided**

½ cup **diced red bell pepper (about ½ a pepper)**

1 cup **diced brown mushrooms**

1 pound **lean ground turkey meat**

½ cup **part-skim ricotta cheese**

1 tablespoon **Dijon mustard**

½ **Fuji apple, peeled and shredded**

⅛ teaspoon **ground black pepper**

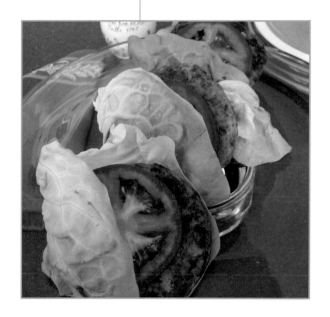

Preparation:

Heat 1 teaspoon of the olive oil on medium heat and lightly sauté peppers, approximately 2 minutes. Add the mushrooms and continue to cook until both are tender, about 6-8 minutes. Put in mixing bowl and set aside to cool. Add ground turkey, ricotta cheese, Dijon mustard, apple and pepper. Mix together and form 4 burgers. Put in refrigerator for 10-15 minutes to set.

Heat the other teaspoon of olive oil in the saucepan, and sauté burgers on one side for 3-4 minutes. Flip over and sauté the other side for 3-4 minutes, using cover. Reduce heat, partially cover with lid and cook until temperature is 160 degrees. Serve immediately.

Recipe and Nutrition Tip:
Ricotta cheese not only increases the calcium content of these burgers, but is a key ingredient in keeping them moist and tender. Inspired by a family friend. Delicate but delicious.

Nutrition Facts	Per Serving
Calories	238
Protein	26 grams
Total Carbohydrates	7 grams
Total Fat	12 grams
Fiber	1 gram
Sodium	210 mg.

Curried Scallops

Servings: 4
Prep Time: 15 mins
Cook Time: 10 mins

Ingredients:

1 pound **dry sea scallops, tough muscle removed (about 12)**

1 teaspoon **curry powder, divided**

1½ tablespoons **butter, divided**

⅓ cup **shallots, thinly sliced**

2 tablespoons **apple cider or rice wine vinegar**

1 **medium sweet tart apple, cored, thinly sliced and diced into tiny pieces**

Salt and pepper to taste

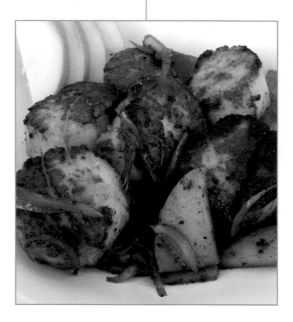

Preparation:

Rinse scallops and pat dry. Toss scallops with small amount of sea salt and pepper and ¼ of the curry powder. Set aside.

Melt 1 tablespoon butter in a large skillet. With tongs, place scallops in pan and sauté approximately 2-3 minutes on each side until seared.

Remove scallops from pan to heated plate. Cover with foil. Add remaining butter, curry powder, shallots, vinegar, and apples to pan. Sauté mixture about 4-6 minutes until apples are soft.

Once apples are soft and liquid is reduced by half, add scallops back to pan to coat. Serve hot.

Recipe Tip:
Dry sea scallops have not been treated or soaked in water, which helps eliminate wetness and promotes a browner exterior.

Nutrition Facts	Per Serving
Calories	153
Protein	19 grams
Total Carbohydrates	6 grams
Total Fat	5 grams
Fiber	.5 grams
Sodium	390 mg.

Tilapia with Caponata

Servings: 2
Prep Time: 5 mins
(not including Caponata)
Cook Time: 6 mins

Ingredients:

½ pound **Tilapia or other white fish**

½ tablespoon **unsalted butter**

1 teaspoon **olive oil**

Juice of 1 lemon (split in 2 parts)

1 cup **Quick and Easy Caponata (see recipe)**

Pinch of salt and pepper to taste

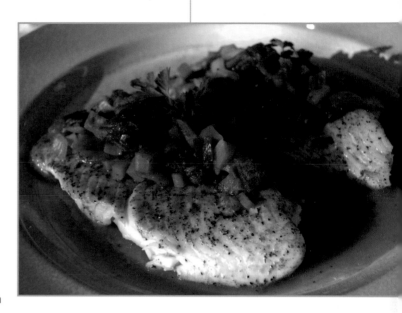

Preparation:

Rinse fish and pat dry. Heat butter and olive oil in saucepan. Squeeze juice of half the lemon on fish and finish with a pinch of salt and pepper. Sauté in medium saucepan about 2-3 minutes per side. Remove from the pan and squeeze with other half of lemon. Top each piece with ½ cup of Caponata.

Recipe and Nutrition Tip:
Any mild white fish can be used in this recipe. The Caponata spices up the fish and adds phytochemicals to your meal.

Nutrition Facts	Per Serving
Calories	200
Protein	24 grams
Total Carbohydrates	9 grams
Total Fat	8 grams
Fiber	3 grams
Sodium	281 mg.

Wild Salmon with Fennel and Orange

Servings: 4
Prep Time: 15 mins
Cook Time: 10-20 mins

Ingredients:

1½ pounds **wild salmon (filleted and skinless)**

Juice of half a lemon

½ **fennel bulb (sliced in ⅛ inch slices) and fronds**

1 tablespoon **fresh grated ginger**

Lemon slices (6-8 large)

1 tablespoon **unsalted butter (broken into pea-sized pieces)**

⅛ teaspoon **red pepper flakes**

Juice of half a naval orange

Recipe and Nutrition Tip:
A beautiful and impressive dish worth the time investment. Leftovers are good on a salad. Wild salmon is high in omega-3 fatty acids.

Nutrition Facts	Per Serving
Calories	281
Protein	4 grams
Total Carbohydrates	4 grams
Total Fat	13 grams
Fiber	1 gram
Sodium	81 mg.

Preparation:

Rinse salmon with juice of half a lemon and pat dry. Lay 1 ½ feet of tin foil, shiny side down, on the counter. Lay fennel slices with some fronds, half of the grated fresh ginger, and half the lemon slices on the tin foil making a bed so the salmon will not touch the tin foil.

Place salmon on the bed with the filleted (edge where the skin was attached) side down. Scatter butter pieces and red pepper flakes on top of salmon. Sprinkle the other half of ginger, lemon slices, and a few slices of fennel and fronds over salmon. Finish with juice of the orange on top.

To make a packet, take the long ends of the tin foil, fold together and seal over fish. Then, take the short ends of the tin foil and fold in to seal.

Grill packets over medium heat 4 to 5 minutes, and flip packet over for another 4 minutes. Remove and invert back over. Open packet and serve.

Variation: Place in oven for 15-20 minutes at 400 degrees or until desired doneness.

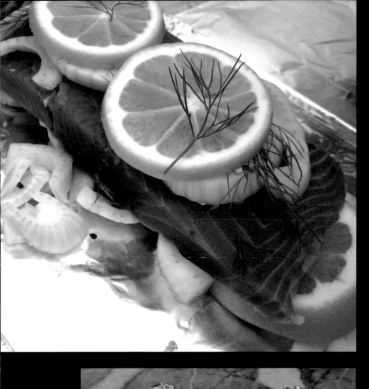

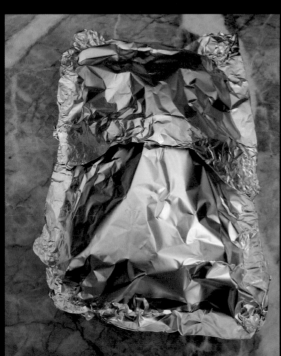

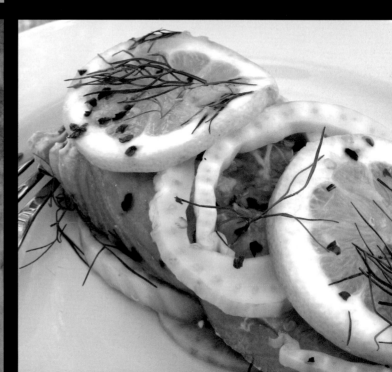

Cinnamon Lamb Chops

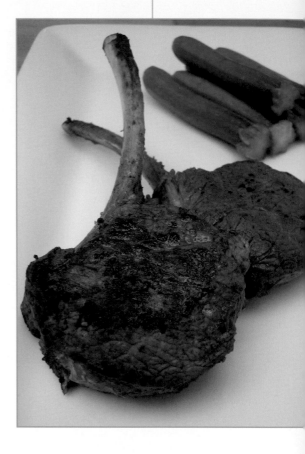

Servings: 4
Prep Time: 6 mins
Cook Time: 10-15 mins

Ingredients:

2 tablespoons **unsalted butter, softened**

1 teaspoon **ground cinnamon**

¼ teaspoon **sea salt**

¼ teaspoon **black pepper**

4 **loin-cut lamb chops (about 3-4 ounces each or 1 pound total)**

Preparation:

Mix butter, cinnamon, salt, and pepper into a paste and rub over both sides of each lamb chop in equal proportions.

Sauté lamb chops in a large dry skillet set over medium heat until browned, about 4-5 minutes per side. Let rest 2 to 3 minutes and serve.

Nutrition Facts	Per Serving
Calories	215
Protein	24 grams
Total Carbohydrates	.5 grams
Total Fat	12.5 grams
Fiber	0 grams
Sodium	198 mg.

Pork Tenderloin with Fennel and Apple

Servings: 4
Prep Time: 20 mins
Cook Time: 45 mins

Ingredients:

1 pound **pork tenderloin, trimmed**

2 tablespoons **olive oil, divided**

2 large **shallots, sliced**

1 medium **sweet-tart apple, Fuji or Pink Lady, cored and thinly sliced**

1 large **fennel bulb, trimmed and thinly sliced**

1 tablespoon **fennel fronds, chopped and divided**

3 tablespoons **apple cider vinegar**

Salt and pepper to taste

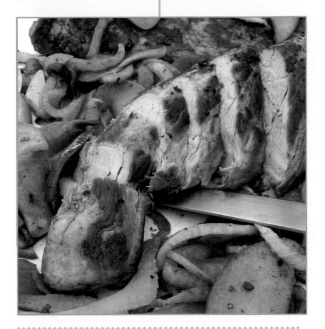

Preparation:

Preheat oven to 475 degrees, position racks to upper and lower thirds of oven.

Rub tenderloin with ½ tablespoon of olive oil and season with salt and pepper to taste. Set aside.

Toss shallots, apples and fennel with 1 tablespoon of oil and place in roasting pan. Place pan on lower rack for approximately 20 minutes, stirring twice until tender.

During roasting of apple mixture:
Heat ½ tablespoon of oil in large oven-proof skillet over medium heat. Sear and brown the pork on each side for two minutes. (Do not force turning the meat, since as it cooks it will easily turn).

Once the pork is browned, transfer the skillet to top rack in oven. Roast until internal temperature registers 145 degrees, approximately 12-15 minutes or barely pink. Transfer meat to plate or cutting board to rest for 10-15 minutes.

Place apple and fennel mixture in skillet. Deglaze pan with 3

Recipe Tip:
A good dish for company that has a nice combination of sour with sweet.

Nutrition Facts	Per Serving
Calories	227
Protein	32 grams
Total Carbohydrates	15 grams
Total Fat	2 grams
Fiber	3 grams
Sodium	98 mg.

tablespoons of vinegar. Slice pork and place on platter. Top with apple and fennel mixture. Garnish with fennel fronds if desired.

Variation: Chop apple and fennel mix similar to a chutney style.

Rosemary Lemon Lamb

Servings: 4
Prep Time: 5 mins
Cook Time: 10 mins

Ingredients:

1 pound **lamb chops, 1½ inches thick**

Juice of one lemon

1 **garlic clove, crushed**

1 tablespoon **fresh rosemary, chopped**

¼ teaspoon **pepper**

⅛ teaspoon **salt**

½ tablespoon **coconut oil**

Recipe and Nutrition Tip:
Remarkably light in taste with complimentary flavors. For best results, be sure not to overcook the lamb.

Nutrition Facts	Per Serving
Calories	182
Protein	24 grams
Total Carbohydrates	1.5 grams
Total Fat	8.5 grams
Fiber	0 grams
Sodium	150 mg.

Preparation:

Trim fat off meat with sharp knife.

Pour lemon juice on meat and let set while making rub.

Make a rub of garlic, rosemary, salt and pepper. Spread rub over both sides of chops.

Heat coconut oil in heavy skillet over medium heat until shimmering. Cook chops on each side for 4-5 minutes or until medium rare to medium.

Hint: To keep lamb chops warm while preparing other items, turn chops on end with bone touching pan only - this will help not to overcook the meat.

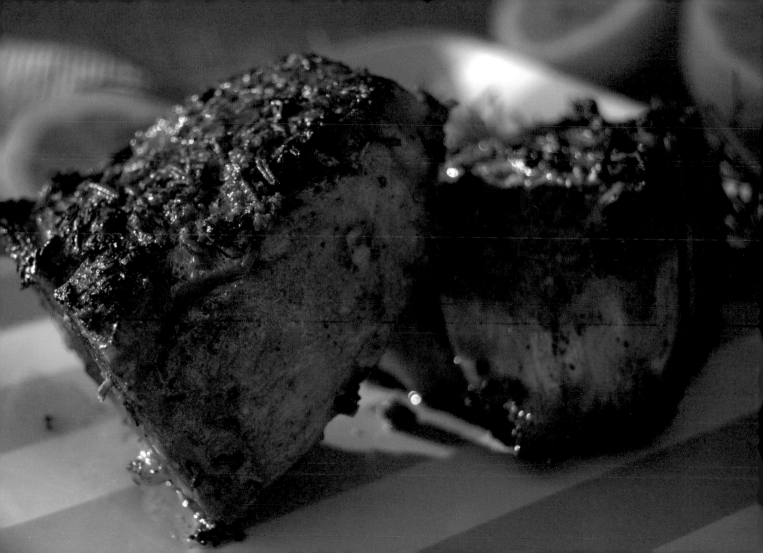

Pork with Apples and Carrots

Servings: 4
Prep Time: 10- 20 mins
Cook Time: 20-25 mins

Ingredients:

4 ½ **boneless skinless pork loins**
(about 1/2 inch thick or 4 ounces each)

1 tablespoon **of olive oil, divided**

1 teaspoon **ground ginger**

½ teaspoon **ground sage**

¼ teaspoon **ground pepper**

1 tablespoon **unsalted butter**

1 **large apple (Pink Lady works well), peeled, cored**
and cubed

1 cup **diced carrots (approximately 5 small)**

¼ cup **water**

Salt and pepper to taste

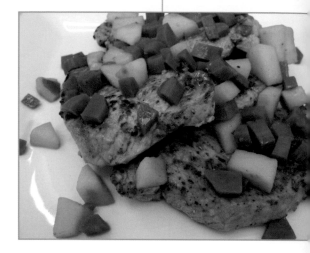

Preparation:

Rub half the oil on all sides of meat. Mix ginger, sage, and pepper together and rub on both sides of pork chops.

Heat the other half of the oil in a large skillet over medium heat. Add pork to the skillet and sauté until brown, about 3-4 minutes per side and then transfer to a platter.

Add butter, chopped apple, and carrots to the skillet and sauté until golden brown. Stir in approximately ¼ cup of water and cook until tender. Add pork back to the skillet and simmer until hot. Season to taste with salt and pepper.

Recipe Tip:
This dish is hearty and can be enjoyed year round. They taste much better than the old tough pork chops you may have had when you were a kid. The spices can be adjusted to taste.

Nutrition Facts	Per Serving
Calories	337
Protein	33 grams
Total Carbohydrates	11 grams
Total Fat	6 grams
Fiber	2 grams
Sodium	90 mg.

Grapefruit and Avocado Salad

Servings: 4 small dinner salads
Prep Time: 10 mins

Ingredients:

One **head butter lettuce**

1 **medium pink grapefruit**

1 **Haas avocado**

1 tablespoon **white balsamic vinegar**

1 tablespoon **apple cider vinegar**

1 tablespoon **olive oil**

Fresh ground pepper to taste

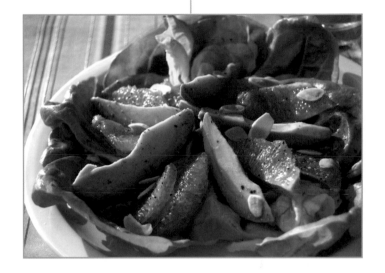

Preparation:

Wash and drain lettuce. Peel grapefruit and cut into sections, removing the white membrane. Peel and slice avocado lengthwise.

Mix vinegars and olive oil in a small bowl. Make a bed of lettuce on plates.

Alternate grapefruit sections and avocado on the lettuce in a pinwheel fashion. Drizzle dressing over salads and top with fresh ground pepper.

Variation: Top with pomegranate seeds or sliced almonds for a festive look.

Nutrition Tip:
Pink grapefruit contain lycopenes, which help in the prevention of prostrate cancer. Avocados are high in monounsaturated fat, which help increase HDL or good cholesterol.

Nutrition Facts	Per Serving
Calories	128
Protein	2 grams
Total Carbohydrates	13 grams
Total Fat	9 grams
Fiber	5.7 grams
Sodium	5 mg.

Avocado Feta and Tomato Salad

Servings: 4 small dinner salads
Prep Time: 20 mins

Ingredients:

2 cups **chopped tomatoes**

1 **Haas avocado, cubed**

½ **cup feta cheese**

1 tablespoon **red wine or rice wine vinegar**

Juice of half a small lemon

Fresh ground pepper to taste

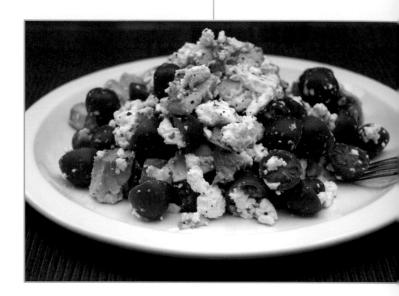

Preparation:

Mix all ingredients together. Cover and let sit in refrigerator for 15 minutes to enhance the flavors.

Recipe Tip:
This salad comes in handy when you don't have lettuce on hand. You need only a few ingredients and less than 5 minutes to add a colorful salad to lunch or dinner.

Nutrition Facts	Per Serving
Calories	124
Protein	4 grams
Total Carbohydrates	8 grams
Total Fat	9 grams
Fiber	3.5 grams
Sodium	216 mg.

Broccoli Ricotta Soup

Servings: 4
Prep Time: 10 mins
Cook Time: 20 mins

Ingredients:

½ tablespoon **extra virgin olive oil**

1 shallot, diced

1 pound **broccoli florets (about 5-6 cups,
cut into small pieces)**

2 cups **low-sodium vegetable broth**

⅛ teaspoon **garlic powder**

1 cup **part-skim ricotta cheese**

Pinch of dried basil

Salt and pepper to taste

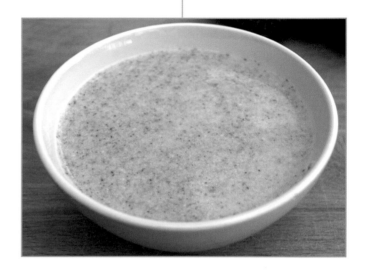

Preparation:

Heat olive oil in saucepan over medium heat. Add shallot and sauté one minute. Add broccoli florets and stir until slightly brown and tender.

Add vegetable broth to saucepan and bring to a boil. Reduce heat and simmer 15-20 minutes until broccoli is tender.

Transfer mixture to blender and puree until slightly chunky. Add ricotta cheese, garlic powder, and basil and puree until smooth. May need to reheat before serving.

Recipe and Nutrition Tip:
Broccoli is a cruciferous vegetable known for its anti-cancer properties, high in vitamins A, C and K in addition to many phytochemicals. This nutrient-packed dish combines broccoli with ricotta cheese to add calcium. Olive oil increases omega-3 and monounsaturated fat.

Nutrition Facts	Per Serving
Calories	159
Protein	13 grams
Total Carbohydrates	11 grams
Total Fat	8 grams
Fiber	3 grams
Sodium	219 mg.

CORE Salad

Servings: 4
Prep Time: 5 mins
Cook Time: 10-15 mins

Ingredient ideas:

Romaine, red or green leaf or other lettuces

Tomatoes, cucumbers or mushrooms

Any fresh vegetables

Hard-boiled eggs

Cheese – hard, parmesan or feta/goat

Leftover chicken, turkey or steak

Nuts or seeds

Leftover cooked vegetables

Cut up fruit (apples, pears, berries or other)

Named by Susan's father (CORE ="Clean out the refrigerator"), this salad is made with whatever you happen to find in your refrigerator. Never the same twice, it changes with each season as to what you have on hand. This is an excellent way to use your leftovers and encourage creativity with your meals.

Preparation:
Mix all ingredients together and enjoy. Use an oil and vinegar dressing or Jeffrey's Salad Dressing.

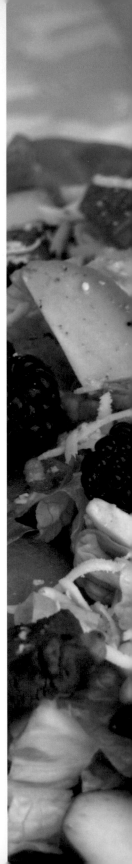

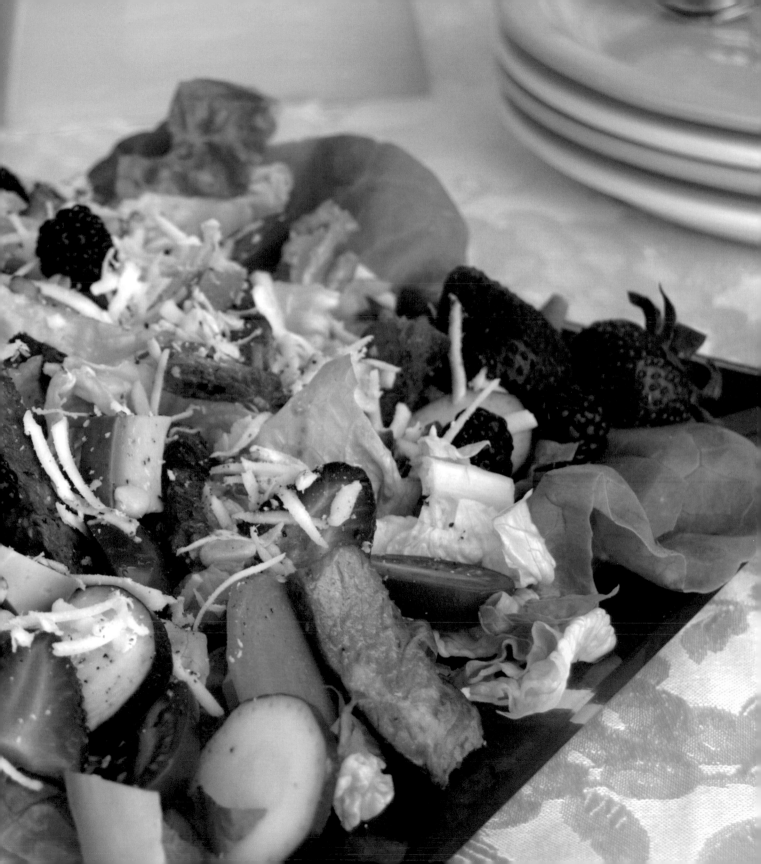

Butternut Squash Soup

Servings: 6
Prep Time: 15 mins
Cook Time: 45 mins

Ingredients:

1 **medium to large butternut squash**

1 tablespoon **unsalted butter**

1 **large shallot, finely chopped**

5 cups **water**

½ cup **1% milk**

1 **pinch cinnamon**

1 **pinch grated nutmeg**

Salt and pepper to taste

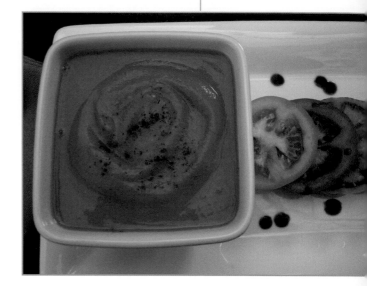

Preparation:

Cut butternut squash lengthwise and scoop out seeds and strings. In a stockpot, heat butter and sauté seeds, strings, and shallots until shallots are translucent. Add water, bring to a boil, and reduce heat.

Place steamer basket in stockpot. Place squash face down in a steamer basket. Cover and steam until tender, approximately 20 to 30 minutes. Remove squash and scrape out the inside flesh, throwing away the skin. In a mesh strainer, strain the seeds, strings and shallots over a bowl, saving the liquid. Rinse out the pot to remove any seeds or strings.

In blender, puree squash and the saved liquid and milk in batches. Put back into pot and add cinnamon and nutmeg. Reheat until hot (do not boil). Add more milk if necessary.

Recipe and Nutrition Tip:
Butternut squash is an excellent source of vitamins A and C, beta-carotene, fiber, potassium and magnesium. A hearty filling soup worth the time it takes to make.

Nutrition Facts	Per Serving
Calories	69
Protein	2 grams
Total Carbohydrates	12 grams
Total Fat	2 grams
Fiber	3 grams
Sodium	15 mg.

Easy Tomato Sauce/Soup

Servings: 6
Prep Time: 15 mins
Cook Time: 25 mins

Ingredients:

For Sauce:

2 tablespoons **minced garlic**

4 tablespoons **minced shallots**

1 teaspoon **olive oil**

2 **14.5-ounce cans low sodium diced tomatoes**

2 cups **low sodium vegetable broth**

2 tablespoons **Italian seasoning**

For Soup:

1½ cups **1% milk**

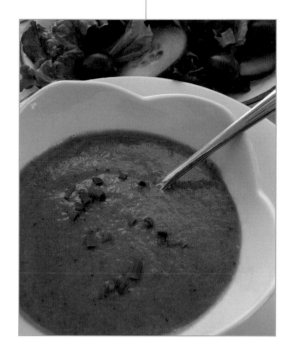

Preparation:

For Sauce:
Dice garlic and shallots. In a small saucepan, heat olive oil. Add shallots and garlic and sauté until tender. Add diced tomatoes, vegetable broth, Italian seasoning, salt and pepper to taste, and bring to a boil. Simmer for 15 to 20 minutes.

For Soup:
Put half of the sauce in blender with ¾ cup of 1% milk and puree. Repeat with other half of sauce with the same amount of milk. Return to pot if necessary to heat before serving. Top with chives or parsley if desired.

Recipe Tip:
Not quite as good as the sauce Susan's mother made that took all day, but a close version and so much easier and time efficient. Good for many of your recipes that call for tomato sauce.

Nutrition Facts	Per Serving
Calories	67/ 97
Protein	1.0/3.5 grams
Total Carbohydrates	8/11 grams
Total Fat	2/ 2.5 grams
Fiber	1.3/ 1.3 grams
Sodium	159/191 mg.

Egg Salad Twist

Ingredients:

4 large eggs

3 tablespoons **chopped celery**

2 tablespoons **plain low fat yogurt**

1 tablespoons **fresh lemon juice**

1½ teaspoons **Dijon mustard**

⅛ teaspoon **black pepper**

⅛ teaspoon **kosher or sea salt**

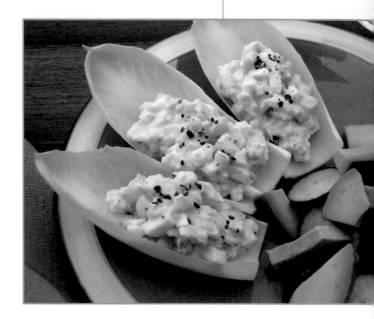

Preparation:

Fill medium saucepan with cold water. Add pinch of salt and eggs, bringing to a boil over high heat.   Once water is boiling, remove from heat and cover. Let rest for 20 minutes. Drain and rinse with cold water. Submerge the eggs in cold water and let set for 10 minutes to stop further cooking.

Remove shells and chop egg to desired consistency.   Mix remaining ingredients into eggs. Serve in butter lettuce or endive, similar to a taco.

Variation: Mix in chopped tomato, avocado, cucumber, scallions or dill pickle.

Nutrition Tip:
Using plain yogurt instead of mayonnaise lowers the fat without compromising on taste. Eggs are the highest quality protein that exists.

Nutrition Facts	Per Serving
Calories	157
Protein	13 grams
Total Carbohydrates	5 grams
Total Fat	9 grams
Fiber	0 grams
Sodium	358 mg.

Jeffrey's Chicken Salad

Servings: 6
Prep Time: 15 mins
Cook Time: 20 mins

Ingredients:

1½ pounds **skinless, boneless chicken breasts**

¼ cup **of plain low fat yogurt**

2 teaspoons **regular mustard**

1 teaspoon **of honey**

½ teaspoon **plus pinch curry powder**

⅛ teaspoon **plus pinch garlic powder**

Pepper to taste

1 **tart red apple (Pink Lady works well), diced**

½ cup **pecans**

¼ cup **unsweetened coconut**

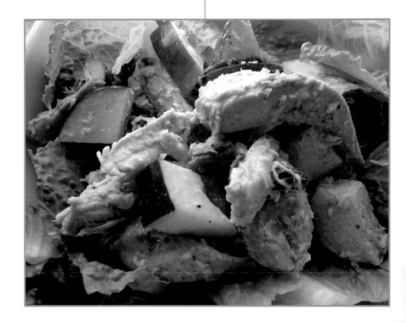

Preparation:

Rinse chicken and boil in medium saucepan with a pinch of sea salt until meat is opaque.

Cube chicken. Combine yogurt, mustard, honey, and spices. Mix in chicken. Add the apple, pecans and coconut. Serve on a bed of lettuce.

Jeffrey's Note:

When I was a little boy my grandmother would make a wonderfully rich chicken salad. I created a modified healthier version, which is a definite staple in our house. Great for lunches.

Nutrition Tip:
Adding apples adds the polyphenol quercetin, thought to lower LDL (bad) cholesterol. The combination of quercetin and the nuts, high in mono-unsaturated fat, provides a health-packed lunch for those with high cholesterol values.

Nutrition Facts	Per Serving
Calories	271
Protein	34 grams
Total Carbohydrates	7 grams
Total Fat	11 grams
Fiber	2 grams
Sodium	88 mg.

"Taco" Salad

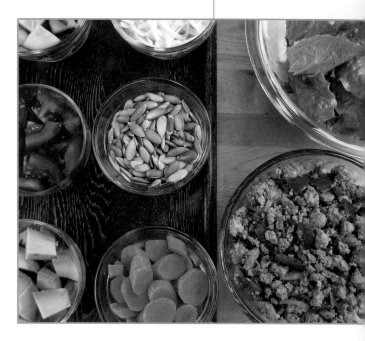

Servings: 6
Prep Time: 15 mins
Cook Time: 15 mins

Ingredients:

1 tablespoon **olive oil**

½ medium **sweet yellow onion, sliced**

1 **large clove garlic, minced**

1 **medium red bell pepper, sliced**

1½ **teaspoons cumin**

1 teaspoon **chili powder**

1 pound **lean ground turkey meat**

1-2 **heads romaine lettuce**

6 tablespoons **grated Monterey Jack cheese**

2 **large tomatoes, diced**

2 **medium carrots, sliced/diced**

½ **medium cucumber, diced**

1 **Haas avocado, sliced**

6 tablespoons **raw, unsalted pumpkin seeds, toasted**

Preparation:

In a medium-sized skillet, sauté onion, garlic and pepper in olive oil over medium heat until tender. Add spices and stir. Mix in turkey and sauté another 5-8 minutes until cooked through.

Wash and dry lettuce and assemble on plates. Top with turkey mixture, cheese, tomatoes, carrots, cucumber, avocado, and pumpkin seeds in six equal portions.

Use salsa, creamy salad dressing, or a little sour cream as desired for dressing.

Recipe and Nutrition Tip:
An easy meal to "assemble" for company, or a way to get young family members involved in cooking. The pumpkin seeds add crunch to the salad as well as being a good source of iron and zinc. Cucumbers and carrots add additional crunch and color.

Nutrition Facts	Per Serving
Calories	321
Protein	20 grams
Total Carbohydrates	13 grams
Total Fat	20 grams
Fiber	6 grams
Sodium	141 mg.

Tangy Tuna Salad

Ingredients:

One **6-ounce can light tuna, drained**

Juice of one medium lemon

1 tablespoon **olive oil**

1 tablespoon **red wine vinegar**

1 medium **cucumber, peeled and diced**

Fresh ground pepper to taste

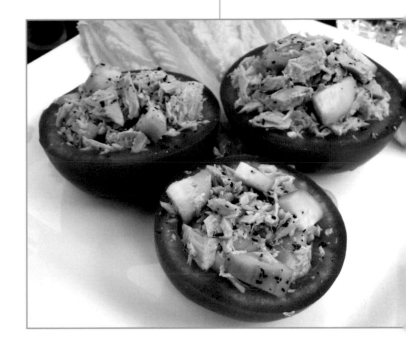

Preparation:

Put tuna in medium bowl and fluff with fork. Mix in remaining ingredients. Enjoy by itself or over lettuce.

Variation: Add diced tomatoes or avocado.

Recipe and Nutrition Tip:
Light tuna has one third less mercury than canned white albacore tuna.

Nutrition Facts	Per Serving
Calories	180
Protein	22 grams
Total Carbohydrates	4 grams
Total Fat	9 grams
Fiber	1 gram
Sodium	290 mg.

Tomato, Cucumber and Dill Salad

Servings: 4 small
dinner salads
Prep Time: 15 mins
(plus 15 mins for refrigeratic

Ingredients:

2 cups **cherry or grape tomatoes, halved**

2 **Persian cucumbers or 1 regular, seeded and peeled**

1 teaspoon **dried dill**

1 tablespoon **red wine vinegar**

1 tablespoon **olive oil**

Fresh ground pepper to taste

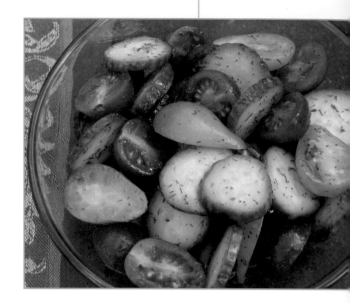

Preparation:

Cube cucumbers and mix with tomatoes.

Stir together dill, vinegar and olive oil and pour mixture over cucumber and tomatoes. Cover and refrigerate for at least 15 minutes to marinate. Serve cold.

Recipe and Nutrition Tip:
Persian cucumbers are handy since they contain no seeds. Their sweet flavor and crunchy watery texture make them a great addition to any salad.

Nutrition Facts	Per Serving
Calories	56
Protein	1 gram
Total Carbohydrates	5 grams
Total Fat	4 grams
Fiber	1.5 grams
Sodium	5 mg.

Sun-Dried Tomato Pesto

Servings: 6 – 2 tbs servings

Ingredients:

1 **garlic clove, chopped**

1 teaspoon **red wine vinegar**

1 **medium shallot, chopped**

2 tablespoons **chopped parsley**

8.5 ounce **jar of sun-dried tomatoes in oil, drained**

¼ cup **macadamia nuts, chopped**

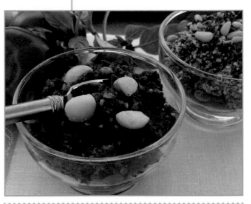

Preparation:

Put all ingredients in a food processor or blender and pulsate until desired consistency. Put on turkey cutlets or chicken breasts and bake, or use as a dip with vegetables. Store in refrigerator.

Nutrition Facts	Per Serving
Calories	68
Protein	1 gram
Total Carbohydrates	4 grams
Total Fat	6 grams
Fiber	1.3 grams
Sodium	34 mg.

Lemon Basil Pesto

Servings: 6 – 1 tbs servings

Ingredients:

1 **garlic clove, chopped**

2 teaspoons **lemon juice**

1 tablespoon **chopped parsley**

1 cup **tightly-packed stemmed basil, chopped**

2 tablespoons **pine nuts**

Pepper to taste

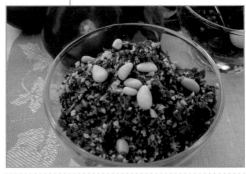

Preparation:

Put all ingredients in a food processor or blender and pulsate until desired consistency

Put on turkey or chicken and bake, or use as a dip with vegetables. Store in refrigerator.

Nutrition Facts	Per Serving
Calories	22
Protein	.6 grams
Total Carbohydrates	1 gram
Total Fat	2 grams
Fiber	.5 grams
Sodium	1 mg.

Jeffrey's Salad Dressing

Servings: 9 – 2 tbs servings
Prep Time: 5 mins

Ingredients:

¼ cup **white balsamic vinegar**

¼ cup **red wine vinegar**

2-3 tablespoons **fresh lemon juice**

¼ teaspoon **black pepper**

¼ teaspoon **garlic powder**

1 tablespoon **Dijon mustard**

2-3 tablespoons **finely-grated parmesan cheese**

2-3 tablespoons **good quality olive oil**

Recipe and Nutrition Tip:
A variation of Susan's Aunt Lydia's salad dressing. Great as both a dressing and marinade. Keeps for a month in a glass container in the refrigerator.

Nutrition Facts	Per Serving
Calories	67
Protein	1 gram
Total Carbohydrates	2 grams
Total Fat	6 grams
Fiber	0 grams
Sodium	77 mg.

Preparation:
Mix together all ingredients and serve on salad. Store remaining dressing in refrigerator. Prior to using, set out for 15 minutes or run container under hot water to melt any oil that turned solid by being refrigerated.

Creamy Salad Dressing

Servings: 6 – 2 tbs servings
Prep Time: 5 mins

Ingredients:

1 tablespoon **plain low fat yogurt**

3 tablespoons **1% milk**

1 tablespoon **Dijon mustard**

¼ teaspoon **dry dill**

½ small **shallot, minced**

½ small **clove garlic, minced**

½ small **cucumber, cut lengthwise and diced**

Recipe and Nutrition Tip:
A good alternative to ranch dressing without the MSG.

Nutrition Facts	Per Serving
Calories	25
Protein	.7 gram
Total Carbohydrates	1.7 grams
Total Fat	1.4 grams
Fiber	0 grams
Sodium	69 mg.

Preparation:
Mix together yogurt, sour cream, milk and mustard. Stir in dill, shallot, garlic, and cucumber. Refrigerate 30 minutes.

Asparagus with Nutmeg

Servings: 4
Prep Time: 2 mins
Cook Time: 5 mins

Ingredients:

1 tablespoon **olive oil**

Asparagus spears, about 20

½ teaspoon **garlic powder**

¼ to ½ teaspoon **fresh-grated nutmeg**

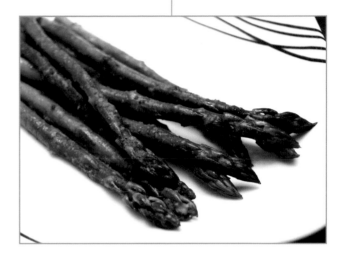

Preparation:

Put olive oil in a large skillet over medium heat. Place prepared asparagus stalks in pan (see tip).

Top asparagus with garlic powder and fresh nutmeg, turning spears to coat. Add 2-3 tablespoons of water to pan and cover. Reduce heat to medium low, and steam spears for approximately 3-4 minutes until desired doneness. Remove and grate additional nutmeg if desired. You may need to add additional water until desired doneness.

Recipe Tip:
To properly store asparagus, snap the woody part of the stalk off (where it naturally breaks off) and place upright in a cup of water in the refrigerator. Change water daily until used (up to 3 days). When choosing asparagus, select ones with spear tips that are closed (i.e. the flowers are not starting to open).

Nutrition Facts	Per Serving
Calories	55
Protein	2 grams
Total Carbohydrates	5 grams
Total Fat	3.5 grams
Fiber	2 grams
Sodium	5 mg.

BBQ Brussels Sprouts

Servings: 8
Prep Time: 20 mins
(plus 1 hr to marinate)
Cook Time: 10 mins

Ingredients:

1 pound **Brussels sprouts**

⅓ cup **Jeffrey's Salad dressing**

or favorite Italian dressing

Preparation:

Clean Brussels sprouts and remove outer leaves. Cut sprouts in half and place in plastic bag with dressing. Marinate in refrigerator for 1 hour.

Grill on BBQ, rotating often for even cooking and browning.

Nutrition Tip:
A wonderful way to enjoy Brussels sprouts without the bitter taste. Brussels sprouts are cruciferous vegetables, high in vitamins C, K and the carotenoid zeaxanthin, helpful in the prevention of age-related macular degeneration.

Nutrition Facts	Per Serving
Calories	45
Protein	2.0 grams
Total Carbohydrates	6 grams
Total Fat	2 grams
Fiber	2 grams
Sodium	41 mg.

Brussels Sprout Hash

Servings: 4
Prep Time: 15 mins
Cook Time: 15 mins

Ingredients:

1 teaspoon **olive oil**

1 medium **chopped shallot**

2 cups **chopped Brussels sprouts**

3 tablespoons **apple cider vinegar**

2 tablespoons **toasted pine nuts**

Ground pepper to taste

Preparation:

Thinly slice shallots and set aside. Shred Brussels sprouts similar to coleslaw. Sauté shallots in the olive oil until translucent, and add Brussels sprouts and sauté until tender.

Once tender, add cider vinegar and remove from heat. Toss with pepper and pine nuts. Serve immediately.

Recipe Tip:
A great dish to share. Your company won't believe they are eating Brussels sprouts!

Nutrition Facts	Per Serving
Calories	62
Protein	2 grams
Total Carbohydrates	5.5 grams
Total Fat	4 grams
Fiber	2 grams
Sodium	14 mg.

Cauliflower Crunch

Servings: 4
Prep Time: 10 mins
Cook Time: 10 mins

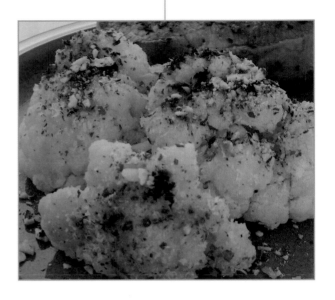

Ingredients:

Large head cauliflower (regular or colorful variety)

1 tablespoon butter, melted

⅓ cup unsweetened coconut

⅓ cup chopped pecans or almonds

Preparation:

Clean and cut cauliflower into flowerets. Place into pot of boiling water and let cook, approximately 2 minutes.

Drain and pat dry. Place florets close together in tin-foiled lined pan and drizzle with butter. Cover with coconut and nuts.

Place under broiler until toasty brown, about 5 to 10 minutes. Important to watch and rotate for even cooking.

Variation: You can microwave cauliflower if short on time.

Recipe Tip:
A great way for children to enjoy vegetables.

Nutrition Facts	Per Serving
Calories	107
Protein	3 grams
Total Carbohydrates	6 grams
Total Fat	8 grams
Fiber	3 grams
Sodium	44 mg.

Cinnamon Butternut Squash

Servings: 4 half-cup serving
Prep Time: 8 mins
Cook Time: 7 mins

Ingredients:

One **medium butternut squash (about 2 cups of squash)**

1½ tablespoons **butter**

1 teaspoon **cinnamon**

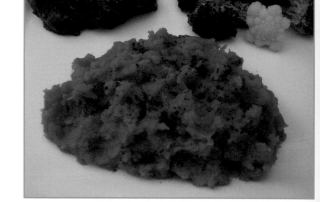

Preparation:

Prepare squash by removing top and bottom. Remove rind with knife or vegetable peeler. Cut squash lengthwise and remove seeds.

Cut squash into medium pieces, rinse and place in a microwavable glass dish. If desired, squash can be steamed on the stove top using a vegetable basket.

Cook for 5-7 minutes until tender when pierced.

Mash with fork or hand masher until consistency of mashed potatoes. Mix in butter and cinnamon.

Variation: You can add toasted pumpkin seeds if desired.

Recipe and Nutrition Tip:
Butternut squash is high in beta carotene, vitamins A, C and fiber. A great dish for children or those who dislike vegetables.

Nutrition Facts	Per Serving
Calories	89
Protein	1 gram
Total Carbohydrates	13.5 grams
Total Fat	4.5 grams
Fiber	4 grams
Sodium	35 mg.

Easy Vegetarian Chili

Servings: 4 1¼ cup servings
Prep Time: 20 mins
Cook Time: 30 mins

Ingredients:

3 **carrots, peeled and diced**

½ **medium yellow onion, chopped**

1 **medium red bell pepper, seeded and chopped**

1 **medium yellow bell pepper, seeded and chopped**

3 teaspoons **chili powder**

1 teaspoon **ground cumin**

1 tablespoon **olive oil**

½ cup **water**

1 14.5-ounce **can low salt diced tomatoes with juice**

1 14-ounce **can dark red kidney beans, rinsed**

1½ cups **of shredded hot pepper Monterey Jack cheese**

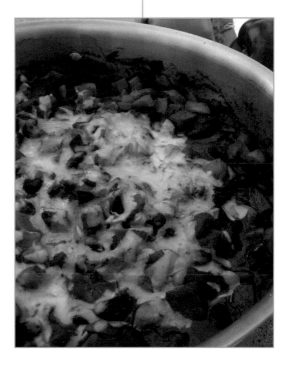

Preparation:

Preheat broiler on low.

Sauté carrots, onions, pepper, chili powder and cumin in olive oil in an oven proof skillet until tender. Add water, tomatoes, and beans. Cook covered for 15 minutes on medium to high heat. Remove cover and stir. Top with cheese and place in broiler until cheese melts.

Garnish with sour cream and lime wedges.

Recipe and Nutrition Tip:
A crunchy colorful dish to make when you need a quick dinner, high in phytochemicals and nutrients. Adjust spices up or down depending on your tastes.

Nutrition Facts	Per Serving
Calories	284
Protein	14 grams
Total Carbohydrates	20 grams
Total Fat	15 grams
Fiber	6 grams
Sodium	447 mg.

Eggplant Parmigiana

Servings: 6
Prep Time: 1 hr
Cook Time: 45 mins

Ingredients:

1 large **eggplant, thinly sliced into medallions with top and bottom removed**

1 **jumbo egg**

1½ **tablespoons olive oil**

Easy Tomato Sauce (see recipe)

10 ounces **part-skim mozzarella cheese, thinly sliced**

2 tablespoons **parmesan cheese**

Salt and pepper to taste

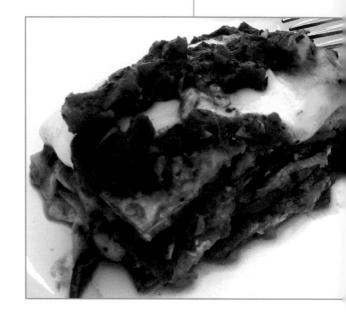

Preparation:

To remove bitter flavor from eggplant, place paper towels between layers of lightly salted eggplant on a cookie sheet. Place a pan filled with water on top of eggplant for 30 minutes to 1 hour. The paper towels will absorb liquid from eggplant.

Dip eggplant in egg and sauté each piece until tender in olive oil. Place eggplant on dry paper towels to soak up any excess oil.

Cover the bottom of a 9x9 baking dish with a thin layer of tomato sauce. Layer eggplant slices (overlapping), followed by a layer of mozzarella cheese, a sprinkling of parmesan cheese, and a thin layer of sauce. Repeat the process until all eggplant and cheese mixtures are used. Serve extra sauce on the side.

Bake in a preheated 350 degree oven for 45 minutes or until bubbling. Remove from oven and let rest for 15 minutes before serving.

Recipe Tip:
An easier version of a traditional elegant Italian dish. Time-consuming, but well worth the effort. A great company dish.

Nutrition Facts	Per Serving
Calories	290
Protein	17 grams
Total Carbohydrates	15 grams
Total Fat	17 grams
Fiber	4 grams
Sodium	688 mg.

Lemon Parmesan Broccoli

Servings: 6
Prep Time: 5 mins
Cook Time: 6 mins

Ingredients:

4 cups broccoli florets

½ cup grated Parmesan cheese

Juice of one medium lemon

2 tablespoons pine nuts

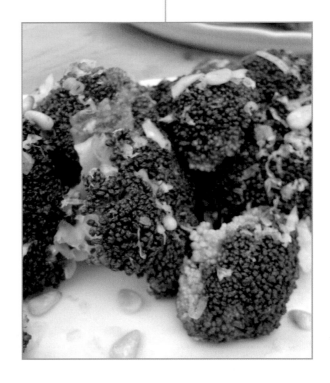

Preparation:

Place florets in microwavable glass dish and heat for 2 ½ minutes on high, or steam for 5-8 minutes on stove. Toss with lemon juice and cheese. Cover for 2 minutes to melt cheese. Top with pine nuts.

Variation: Toast pine nuts for a nutty flavor.

Recipe and Nutrition Tip:
Broccoli is high in vitamins A and C and carotenoids. The cheese contains fat, which helps with absorption of the nutrients in broccoli in addition to increasing the calcium content.

Nutrition Facts	Per Serving
Calories	84
Protein	6 grams
Total Carbohydrates	3.5 grams
Total Fat	5 grams
Fiber	1.5 grams
Sodium	172 mg.

Quick and Easy Caponata

Servings: 10 ½ cup ser
Prep Time: 15 mins
Cook Time: 25 mins

Ingredients:

1 teaspoon **olive oil**

3 **medium carrots, diced**

1 **medium red bell pepper, diced**

1 **medium shallot, chopped**

1 **medium eggplant, diced**

One **14.5-ounce can of diced low-sodium tomatoes with juice**

⅓ teaspoon **ground oregano**

½ cup **red wine vinegar**

Salt and pepper to taste

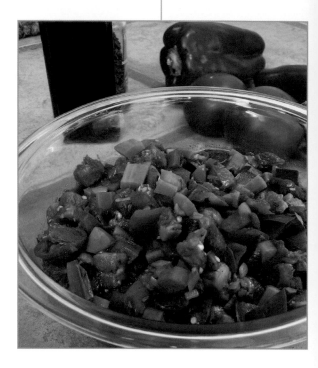

Preparation:

Sauté carrots and red bell pepper in olive oil in a heavy saucepan. Once soft, add shallot and eggplant to mixture. Continue to cook until eggplant becomes tender. Add tomatoes, oregano and vinegar. Bring to boil and simmer for 20-30 minutes. Excellent served hot over fish or poultry or as a side dish.

Variation: You can add a tablespoon of unsweetened dried fruit if desired, such as cranberries.

Recipe and Nutrition Tip:
A beautiful, tangy topping for fish in addition to being a good side dish to spice up meals. High in vitamin C, and beta-carotene.

Nutrition Facts	Per Serving
Calories	38
Protein	1.gram
Total Carbohydrates	7 grams
Total Fat	.6 grams
Fiber	3 grams
Sodium	29 mg.

Vegetable Casserole

Servings: 6
Prep Time: 40 mins
Cook Time: 20 mins

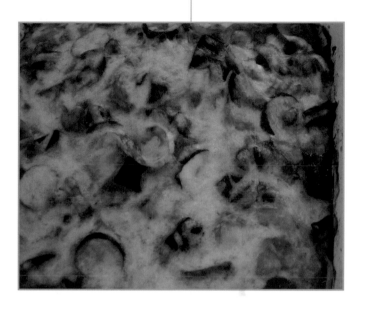

Ingredients:

1 **medium sweet yellow onion, chopped**

1 **medium red bell pepper, chopped**

1½ **tablespoons olive oil**

3 **cloves garlic, minced**

2 **small to medium zucchini, chopped**

1 **medium to large eggplant, cut into 1-inch cubes**

1 cup **tomato puree**

2 **large eggs, beaten**

1 cup **shredded Monterey Jack or mozzarella cheese, divided**

½ cup **shredded parmesan cheese**

Salt and pepper to taste

Preparation:

Preheat oven to 400 degrees.

In a large skillet over medium heat, sauté onions and peppers in olive oil until tender. Add garlic and zucchini and sauté for an additional 4 minutes. Add eggplant, salt and pepper to taste and sauté another 10-15 minutes.

Remove from heat and stir in tomato puree. Stir in beaten eggs, Parmesan cheese and half of Monterey Jack or mozzarella cheese. Pour in a 9 x 9 glass square baking dish, and top with remaining cheese.

Bake for 20-25 minutes. Remove from oven and let rest for 10 minutes before serving.

Variation: Add 1 pound of cooked ground turkey to increase protein.

Recipe Tip:
Simple to increase protein by adding ground turkey, but a great, tasty vegetarian entree or side dish. Good for families or to take to a friend's home.

Nutrition Facts	Per Serving
Calories	207
Protein	11 grams
Total Carbohydrates	13 grams
Total Fat	13 grams
Fiber	5 grams
Sodium	251 grams

Easy and Elegant Frittata

Servings: 8
Prep Time: 20 mins
Cook Time: 25 mins

Ingredients:

½ **sweet yellow medium-sized onion, chopped**

5 cups **chopped vegetables (zucchini, yellow squash, mushrooms, red bell pepper, tomatoes)**

12 **large eggs**

1 tablespoon **olive oil**

2 cups **shredded mozzarella cheese**

2-3 tablespoons **1% milk**

1 tablespoon **Herbs de Provence (or favorite spice)**

¼ teaspoon **garlic powder**

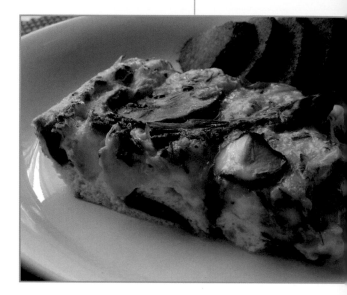

Preparation:

In a medium saucepan, sauté onions and red bell peppers in olive oil until tender for 5 minutes. Add other vegetables and sauté until tender. Remove from heat and set aside.

In a bowl, whisk eggs and add shredded cheese, milk, and spices. Fold in vegetables. Pour mixture into large glass baking dish (9 x 12) and bake at 350 degrees for half an hour or until lightly brown on top and firm. Remove and let rest for 10 minutes. Cut in squares and serve.

Variation: Heirloom tomatoes, broccoli, and asparagus work well for color and taste.

Recipe Tip:
An easy dish to make on the weekends and heat up during the week for breakfast. Frittatas can be made different each time by varying the vegetables. If short on time, eliminate sautéing step, and add all ingredients together and bake.

Nutrition Facts	Per Serving
Calories	209
Protein	18 grams
Total Carbohydrates	6 grams
Total Fat	12 grams
Fiber	1 gram
Sodium	301 mg.

Leftover Feast by Marc Nathanson

Servings: 4
Prep Time: 15 mins
Cook Time: 15 mins

Ingredients:

1 tablespoon **extra-virgin olive oil**

½ **medium size yellow sweet onion, chopped**

1 cup **leftover skinless chicken breasts**

1 cup **leftover lean steak**

2 tablespoons **pine nuts, toasted**

¼ cup **almond quarters or slices, toasted**

1 teaspoon **Italian spice**

½ teaspoon **garlic powder**

1½ cups **bean sprouts**

½ cup **thinly sliced red or orange bell peppers**

1 cup **cubed zucchini or other leftover vegetables**

3 **large eggs, mixed with a little water**

Salt and pepper to taste

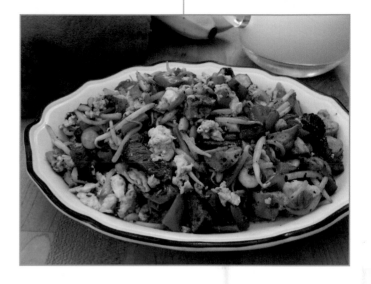

Preparation:

Heat the oil in a large skillet over medium heat. When the oil is hot, add the onions and cook until golden brown, about 2 to 3 minutes. Add chicken, steak, nuts and seasonings, and cook for another 3-4 minutes, stirring frequently.

While continuing to stir, add the bean sprouts and other vegetables, and cook another 2 minutes. Add the egg mixture. Gradually turn eggs, so they are absorbed with the other ingredients. Cover and turn every minute for 4 minutes. Serve hot.

Recipe and Nutrition Tip:
This recipe is a slight variation from Marc's original recipe but incredibly delicious and a great "CORE" dish. Omit eggs for a nice stir fry dish or for a topping for salads.

Nutrition Facts	Per Serving
Calories	275
Protein	25 grams
Total Carbohydrates	8 grams
Total Fat	16 grams
Fiber	3 grams
Sodium	86 mg.

Marc's Note: This recipe, which uses leftovers, was invented for our three kids — Nicole, Adam and David —when they were young. I used to make Sunday breakfast for the family by combining the ingredients left in the refrigerator from the previous week. I am diabetic, so even though the contents would vary somewhat week to week, I chose ingredients low in carbohydrates.

Pizza Eggs

Servings: 2
Prep Time: 5 mins
Cook Time: 5 mins

Ingredients:

2 tablespoons **red bell pepper, diced**

1 teaspoon **olive oil**

4 **medium mushrooms, sliced**

4 **large eggs, beaten with 1 tablespoon water**

Pinch **of oregano**

¼ cup **shredded mozzarella cheese**

Salt and pepper to taste

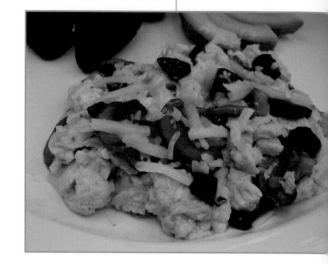

Preparation:

In medium skillet, sauté red bell pepper with olive oil on medium heat for 2–4 minutes or until tender. Add mushrooms and continue to stir until tender. Add in beaten egg mixture and oregano.

With heat resistant spatula, scrape sides of pan often to pull the egg mixture toward the center for even cooking. Once the eggs appear set, add cheese and continue to cook until desired consistency.

Recipe and Nutrition Tip:
Missing pizza? These eggs give you the taste of pizza without all the carbohydrates. Great for a children's breakfast.

Nutrition Facts	Per Serving
Calories	204
Protein	16.5 grams
Total Carbohydrates	4 grams
Total Fat	13 grams
Fiber	.2 grams
Sodium	232 mg.

Ricotta Buckwheat Pancakes

Servings: 20 medium-sized pancakes
Prep Time: 10 mins
(plus 1 hr refrigeration)
Cook Time: 15 mins

Ingredients:

4 **large eggs, separated**

2 cups **part-skim ricotta cheese**

½ cup **buckwheat flour**

¼ teaspoon **salt**

1 tablespoon **sugar**

¾ cup **1% milk**

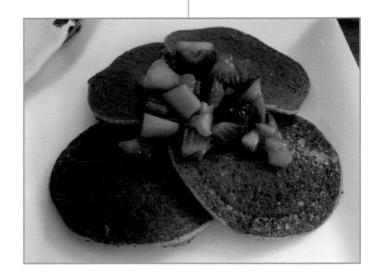

Preparation:

Separate egg whites in a small bowl and yolks in a medium bowl. Set egg whites aside. Mix yolks and ricotta cheese until thoroughly combined. Add the flour, salt and sugar into yolk mixture. Stir the milk.

Beat egg whites with electric mixer until soft peaks form. Gently fold egg whites into yolk mixture. Refrigerate for at least 1 hour or overnight for best results.

Heat griddle with a small amount of butter. Measure batter in approximately ¼ cup increments and pour on hot griddle. Once bubbles start appearing (about 2-3 minutes), gently flip pancake until the other side becomes golden brown (an additional 1-2 minutes). Top with fruit or applesauce.

Tip: Recipe can be halved.

Recipe and Nutrition Tip:

Buckwheat comes from the beet family so it is technically a fruit and not a grain. That makes these pancakes not only a great choice for those with insulin resistance, but also gluten intolerance. High in protein and calcium, a great way for carb lovers to feel spoiled. Very light compared to regular pancakes. The apple blueberry compote makes a great topping.

Nutrition Facts	Per Serving
Calories	66
Protein	5 grams
Total Carbohydrates	3.7 grams
Total Fat	3 grams
Fiber	.5 grams
Sodium	74 mg.

Zucchini and Eggs
(AKA Goo Gooze Eggs)

Servings: 2
Prep Time: 10 mins
Cook Time: 10 mins

Ingredients:

¼ **cup chopped shallots (about 2 medium shallots)**
or ¼ **medium yellow sweet onion**

1 medium **zucchini squash, cut in slices (about 1 cup)**

1 teaspoon **olive oil**

¼ teaspoon **garlic powder**

4 **large eggs**

2 tablespoons **water**

Pepper to taste

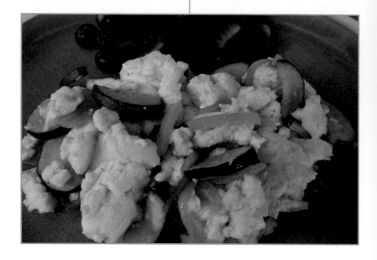

Preparation:

In a medium skillet, sauté shallots and zucchini in 1 teaspoon of olive oil over medium heat until tender. Sprinkle with pepper and garlic powder. Reduce heat.

Whisk eggs with 2 tablespoons of water. Pour in pan and sauté until desired doneness.

*Can be doubled.

Recipe Tip:
Susan's aunt Lydia in N.J. introduced this old Italian dish to us the day she first met Jeffrey. We have made it in our home ever since. Also makes a nice weekend lunch or dinner.

Nutrition Facts	Per Serving
Calories	178
Protein	13 grams
Total Carbohydrates	5 grams
Total Fat	11 grams
Fiber	.5 grams
Sodium	132 mg.

Apple Blueberry Compote

Servings: 6 ½ cup servings
Prep Time: 10 mins
Cook Time: 30 mins

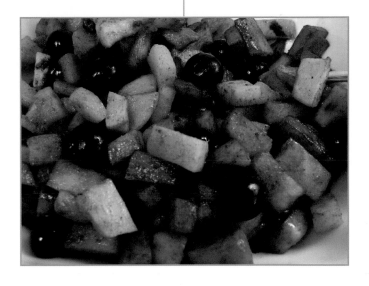

Ingredients:

4 medium **apples, peeled and diced
(mix of Golden Ginger, Gala, Pink Lady, and Fuji)**

1 cup **fresh or frozen blueberries**

¼ teaspoon **cinnamon**

⅛ teaspoon **freshly grated nutmeg**

1 tablespoon **butter, cut in little pieces**

Preparation:
Preheat oven 400 degrees.

Mix apples, blueberries and spices in glass dish. Dot with butter. Bake for 30 minutes. Remove and then stir. Mixture will turn purple with stirring

Variation: Add Healthy Nut Mix for a nice crunch.

Recipe and Nutrition Tip:
We needed a dessert to make with apples and ended up creating this simple recipe by mistake. A great topper for yogurt or cottage cheese. Our cousin, Barbara, prefers this dish to traditional cranberry sauce at holiday meals.

Nutrition Facts	Per Serving
Calories	85
Protein	0 grams
Total Carbohydrates	18 grams
Total Fat	2 grams
Fiber	4 grams
Sodium	0 mg.

Blueberry Peach "Cobbler"

Servings: 4
Prep Time: 10 mins
Cook Time: 20 mins

Ingredients:

3 medium peaches, peeled and sliced

1 cup fresh blueberries

3 tablespoons steel-cut oats

¼ teaspoon fresh ground nutmeg

¼ teaspoon ground cinnamon

Preparation:

Mix together all ingredients. Bake in 400 degree oven for 20 minutes until tender. Serve warm.

Variation: Omit steel-cut oats and add 3 tablespoons of Healthy Nut Mix

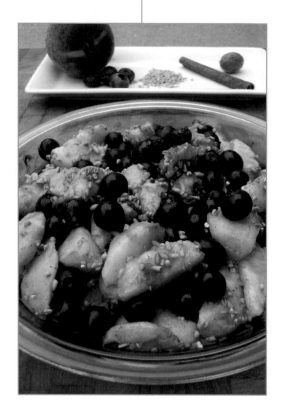

Recipe and Nutrition Tip:
A yummy "cobbler" type of dessert made with steel-cut oats, a better source of whole grains than rolled oats.

Nutrition Facts	Per Serving
Calories	92
Protein	2.5 grams
Total Carbohydrates	21 grams
Total Fat	1 gram
Fiber	3.5 grams
Sodium	5 mg.

Healthy Nut Mix

Servings: 10-¼ cup servings
Prep Time: 10 mins
Cook Time: 15 mins

Ingredients:

¼ cup **raw steel-cut oats**

½ cup **raw pumpkin seeds**

½ cup **coarsely chopped raw cashews**

¼ cup **raw sunflower seeds**

¼ cup **unsweetened dried coconut**

¼ cup **sliced raw almonds**

1 teaspoon **ground cinnamon**

1½ tablespoons **extra virgin coconut oil**

1 teaspoon **honey**

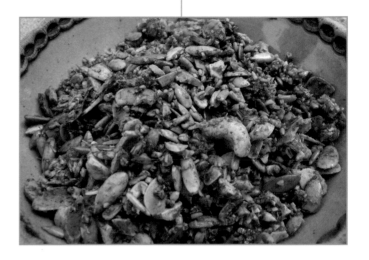

Preparation:

Mix all dry ingredients together. Mix in coconut oil and honey. Spread on cookie sheet and bake at 350 degrees until golden brown, approximately 10-15 minutes, stirring once through the cooking process. Remove from oven and let cool on cookie sheet.

Store in airtight container for up to 5 days or in the freezer for 1 month.

Recipe and Nutrition Tip:
Enjoy as tasty topper for plain yogurt or cottage cheese or as is. Our healthy version of "granola." Coconut oil is high in lauric acid, which is a powerful immune stimulant.

Nutrition Facts	Per Serving
Calories	156
Protein	5 grams
Total Carbohydrates	8 grams
Total Fat	12 grams
Fiber	2 grams
Sodium	2.5 mg.

Hummus 101

Servings: 8-¼ cup servings
Prep Time: 5 mins
            (plus refrigeration time)

Ingredients:

1 **15-ounce can garbanzo beans, drained**

2 tablespoons **fresh lemon juice**

1 tablespoon **olive oil**

¾ teaspoon **garlic powder**

½ teaspoon **ground cumin**

Salt and pepper to taste

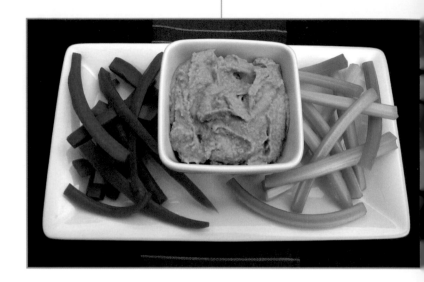

Preparation:

In a food processor, add garbanzo beans, lemon juice, and oil and pulsate until smooth. Add spices to taste and continue to pulsate until well mixed.

Refrigerate for at least 30 minutes prior to eating. Keeps for at least 1 week in the refrigerator.

Recipe Tip:
Not the traditional kind, but a quick, healthy version.

Nutrition Facts	Per Serving
Calories	64
Protein	2.6 grams
Total Carbohydrates	8 grams
Total Fat	2.4 grams
Fiber	2 grams
Sodium	160 mg.

Quick Chocolate Berry Mousse

Servings: 4
Prep Time: 10 mins
(plus refrigeration time)

Ingredients:

1 cup **good quality semi-sweet chocolate chips**

¾ cup **water**

1 tablespoon **100% cane sugar**

½ teaspoon **espresso powder**

3 **egg whites (large to jumbo)**

¼ cup **whipping cream**

4 tablespoons **raspberries, blueberries or blackberries as garnish**

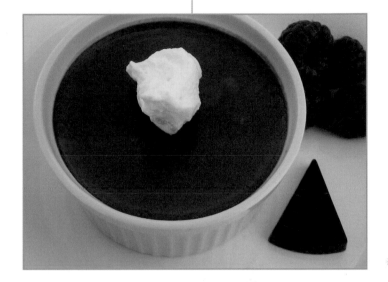

Preparation:

Put chocolate chips in blender or small food processor. Bring water, sugar, and espresso powder to a simmer on the stove. Pour over chocolate chips and blend for 15 seconds. Pour in egg whites* and blend on medium to high speed for one minute.

Pour into 4 ramekins and let chill for at least 2 hours in refrigerator.

Whip cream and put 1 tablespoon on each ramekin. Top with 1 tablespoon of berries.

Recipe and Nutrition Tip:
An easy dessert to make ahead of time for company without too many carbohydrates or calories.

*Heating the water ensures the eggs are safe to eat.

Nutrition Facts	Per Serving
Calories	270
Protein	5 grams
Total Carbohydrates	30 grams
Total Fat	17 grams
Fiber	3 grams
Sodium	53 mg.

Ricotta with Berries

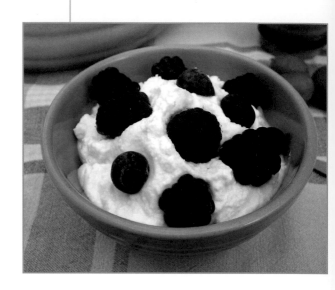

Ingredients:

2 cups **part-skim ricotta cheese**

⅓ cup **sour cream**

1 tablespoon **honey**

¼ -½ teaspoon **vanilla extract (depending on taste preference)**

3 cups **mixed berries (blackberries, strawberries, raspberries, blueberries)**

Preparation:

Mix ricotta cheese, sour cream, honey and vanilla until combined. Refrigerate at least 1 hour until firm.

Spoon into ramekins and top with berries.

Recipe and Nutrition Tip:
If you can find fresh ricotta cheese, this dish is superb. Ricotta has 360 mg. of calcium per half cup, which makes this a high calcium, high-protein dessert.

Nutrition Facts	Per Serving
Calories	227
Protein	14 grams
Total Carbohydrates	14 grams
Total Fat	12 grams
Fiber	3 grams
Sodium	126 mg.

Simple Applesauce

Servings: 6-½ cup servings
Prep Time: 20 mins
Cook Time: 20 mins

Ingredients:

4 cups **peeled, chopped apples**

(about 4-5 medium apples)

1 cup **water**

1 tablespoon **unsalted butter**

½ tablespoon **honey**

¼ teaspoon **cinnamon**

⅛ teaspoon **ground nutmeg**

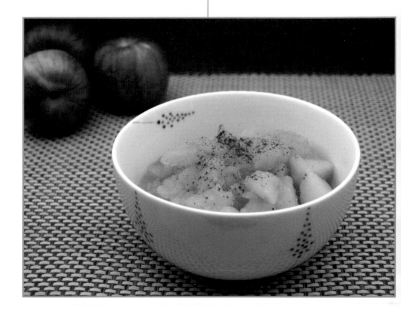

Preparation:

In a quart saucepan over medium heat, place apples in water with lid and cook for 20 minutes until tender, stirring occasionally.

Once apples are at desired consistency, remove from heat and stir in remaining ingredients. Store in refrigerator.

Recipe Tip:
An easy side dish to have on hand to accompany meals or have as a snack with yogurt or cheese. Keeps in the refrigerator for up to 1 week.

Nutrition Facts	Per Serving
Calories	76
Protein	0 grams
Total Carbohydrates	16 grams
Total Fat	2 grams
Fiber	3.5 grams
Sodium	0 mg.

Spiced Pecans

Servings: 10-¼ cup servings
Prep Time: 10 mins
Cook Time: 10 mins

Ingredients:

1 tablespoon **butter**

1½ cups **raw pecan halves**

½ teaspoon **chili powder**

⅛ teaspoon **ground black pepper**

Preparation:

Preheat oven to 350 degrees. In medium skillet, melt butter over medium heat. Stir in chili powder and black pepper. Remove from heat and stir in pecans until completely coated with mixture. Transfer nuts to baking sheet and bake until golden brown, about 8-10 minutes.

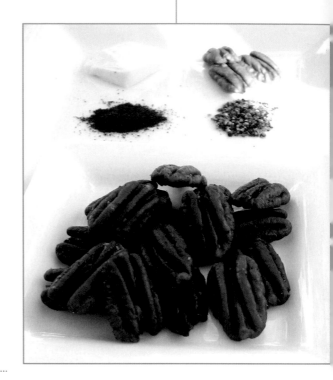

Toasted Nuts or Seeds

These are excellent snacks, and add a variety to other foods. You can create a variety of options as snacks or additions to meals and salads.

Ingredients:

Place 1-2 cups of your favorite nuts or seeds (cashews, pine nuts, almonds, pecans, pumpkin seeds, etc.) in a non-stick skillet (no oil needed). Nuts have natural oil so it is not necessary to add butter for browning. Continually stir over medium heat for even cooking until toasted.

Variation: While nuts are toasting you can add spices, such as cinnamon, garlic, cumin, or allspice.

Recipe and Nutrition Tip:
A great way to spice up veggies, salads or just have as a snack. Goes well on the spiced yams. Nuts are high in monounsaturated fats and satiate your appetite more than other snacks.

Nutrition Facts	Per Serving
Calories	134
Protein	1.6 grams
Total Carbohydrates	2.5 grams
Total Fat	14 grams
Fiber	1.7 grams
Sodium	10 mg.

Healthy Hearty Stuffing

Servings: 15
Prep Time: 30 mins
Cook Time: 45 mins

Ingredients:

8 cups (about 1 pound) grainy wheat bread, torn into bite sizedchunks, stale or lightly toasted

2½ tablespoons butter, divided

1 pound sweet Italian sausage

1 large yellow onion, diced

4 celery stalks, diced

4 cloves garlic, minced

1 green apple, cored and chopped

1 tart red apple, cored and chopped

½ teaspoon ground black pepper

1 tablespoon each fresh thyme, marjoram, and sage, chopped finely, or 1 teaspoon dried of each

4 large eggs

¾ cup low salt chicken broth

6 dried dates, chopped

2 persimmons, peeled and chopped

1 cup chopped toasted pecans

1 teaspoon sea salt

1 cup fresh Italian parsley, finely chopped

Preparation:

Preheat oven to 400 degrees. Grease 9x13 glass baking dish with ½ tablespoon of butter.

Put bread crumbs in large mixing bowl.

Remove sausage from casing and brown in heavy skillet until cooked thoroughly. Remove with slotted spoon and put in the mixing bowl with bread.

Remove excess fat from skillet. Add 2 tablespoons of butter, onion, and celery and sauté for 5 minutes. Add garlic and continue to cook until tender. Add apples, ground pepper, thyme, marjoram and sage and continue to cook for an additional 2 minutes, stirring throughout. Remove from heat and let cool for 5 minutes.

Mix eggs in a large glass measuring cup with the chicken stock. Pour the cooked apple/onion/celery season mixture into the bowl with bread crumbs and sausage. Add dates, persimmons and nuts. Thoroughly stir and add in salt.

Add the egg and broth mixture and mix with large spoon or hands. Stir in parsley. Pour into buttered dish and cover with tin foil. Bake for 25 minutes. Remove foil and continue to bake an additional 15 minutes.

Recipe Tip:
The Japanese persimmons and fresh herbs make this dish quite colorful. This version is a higher in nutrients and fiber than traditional stuffing.

Nutrition Facts	Per Serving
Calories	258
Protein	11 grams
Total Carbohydrates	28 grams
Total Fat	12 grams
Fiber	5 grams
Sodium	522 mg.

Pumpkin Custard

Ingredients:

1½ cups **canned pumpkin**

¼ cup **plain yogurt**

¼ cup **whole milk ricotta cheese**

3 tablespoons **honey**

1 teaspoon **ground cinnamon**

⅛ teaspoon **ground ginger**

⅛ teaspoon **ground allspice**

2 **large eggs, separated**

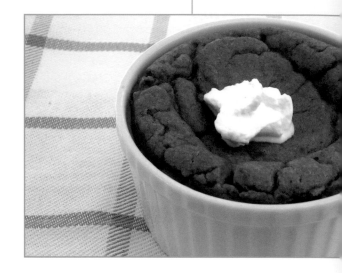

Preparation:

Preheat oven to 350 degrees.

In a medium mixing bowl, stir together canned pumpkin, yogurt and ricotta cheese until blended. Stir in honey and spices.

Separate egg yolks from whites and stir egg yolks into pumpkin mixture. Beat egg whites until stiff peaks form and fold into mixture.

Pour into 6 ramekins and bake at 350 degrees 25-30 minutes until puffed and rounded. Serve immediately.

Variation: May put a dollop of whipped cream on each ramekin.

Recipe and Nutrition Tip:
A great way to enjoy pumpkin "pie" without the extra carbs or calories year round. Pumpkin is high in carotenoids, which are helpful in disease prevention.

Nutrition Facts	Per Serving
Calories	103
Protein	5 grams
Total Carbohydrates	14 grams
Total Fat	3 grams
Fiber	2.7 grams
Sodium	40 mg.

Spiced Yams

Servings: 4
Prep Time: 20 mins
Cook Time: 30 mins

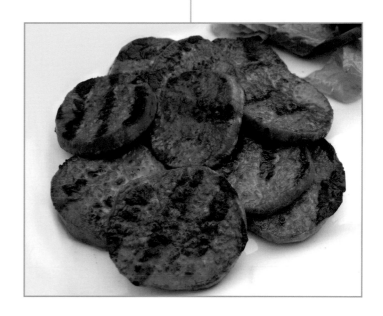

Ingredients:

2 medium yams

2 tablespoons of unsalted butter, melted

1 tablespoon of olive oil

½ tsp. of cinnamon

Pinch of ground ginger

Pinch of ground allspice

Preparation:

Preheat oven to 350 degrees.

Peel yams and slice into 1/4 inch medallions. On a grill pan over medium heat cook yams on both sides until hash marks appear, approximately 2-3 minutes per side.

Mix all other ingredients in a small bowl. When yams are slightly soft, put in glass dish and cover with butter and spice mixture. Place in oven for 10-15 minutes and serve warm.

Recipe and Nutrition Tip:
Yams are a nutrient dense food high in vitamins B6 and C, fiber and potassium. A surprisingly easy and tasty way to enjoy a traditional Thanksgiving dish year round.

Nutrition Facts	Per Serving
Calories	141
Protein	1 gram
Total Carbohydrates	13 grams
Total Fat	9 grams
Fiber	2 grams
Sodium	21 mg.

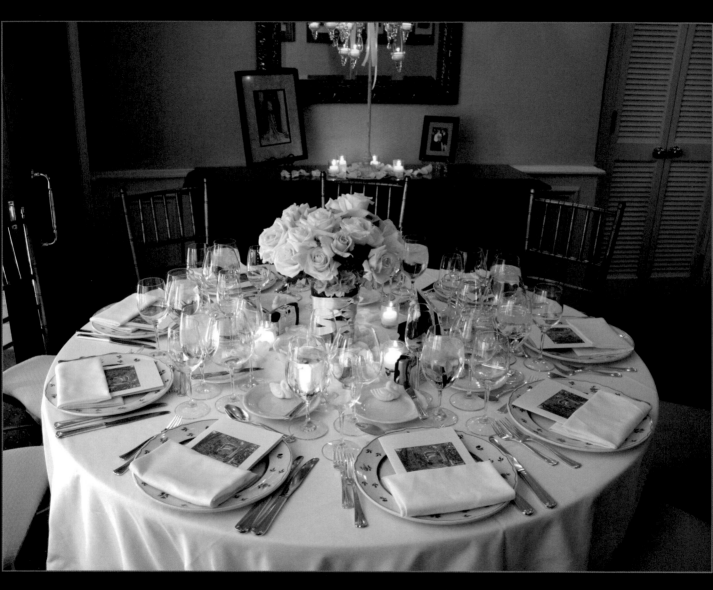

"One cannot think well, love well, sleep well, if one has not dined well."

Part Seven

Optimizing your Longevity and Health

Exercise: Preventive Medicine

It's been a known fact for many years that exercise cures and prevents a substantial number of ailments. Even so, many people did not grow up with exercise as an essential part of their family life. It was only something to do if they had spare time. Historically, and even currently, exercise is not a high priority for a lot of people, which is surprising given the benefits of keeping your body moving.

Present day research confirms that only half of the American population achieves the minimum amount of recommended moderate exercise, and about 40 percent are completely sedentary. This leaves about 10 percent of the population exercising – ranging from moderate exercise to intense exercise. These statistics are inexplicable. Exercise is vastly under valued. Being physically active is the bridge between disease and health.

How did this lack of activity become such an epidemic in America? We know our country was built on hard work. People expended hours and hours of energy engaging in manual labor to survive. You may remember your parents or grandparents saying, "I had to walk to school two miles in the snow, up hill both ways!" Many of us

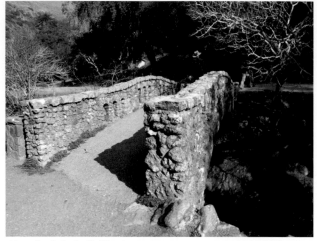

Alum Rock Park, California

have heard this statement and probably smiled, but in pondering this … it is an analogy for what has transpired in our society.

Today's children and teens are usually driven to school and to their after-school activities. Only a few walk or ride their bikes. Furthermore, most adults drive to work unless they live in Manhattan or another walking city. Manual labor has been replaced by machines.   We have appliances at home that do the physical work for us. We hire people to wash our cars, mow our lawns, plant gardens, walk our dogs, and so much more.

A large percentage of the population returns home from work to sit in front of their televisions or computers, go to bed, and wonder why they are feeling lousy and gaining weight.

We have overlooked our need to move, circulate our blood, develop muscles and build strong bones for a good and healthy life. We were built to move.

You Don't Have Time NOT to Exercise

Research confirms that even if a person never lost a pound from exercising, the internal results are well worth the effort. A multitude of studies have also revealed that exercise can deter or eliminate diabetes, atherosclerosis and lower insulin levels, which can decrease the incidence of cancer! Furthermore, the mental health benefits of exercise contribute significantly to emotional stability and a sense of well-being.

Studies give solid evidence that exercise reaps huge rewards. Even a daily walk offers benefits by:

- Increasing the percentage of REM sleep which can increase energy and vitality during the day, allowing you to accomplish more than you could if you had not exercised

- Lowering heart disease by at least 30 percent

- Decreasing the rate of cancer by 35 percent

- Elevating mood by 30 to 50 percent

- Lowering or eliminating Alzheimer's disease, Parkinson's disease and strokes

It sounds too good to be true, but it is!

Individuals who train and exercise at a high level can have up to 50 percent higher protection against viruses, thanks to natural killer cells their bodies generate. At a sports nutrition conference I attended, Professor David Nieman of Appalachian

State University affirmed that near daily exercise creates a cumulative effect on the immune system. His statistics gave evidence - subjects walking moderately for 40 minutes per day have half as many colds or sore throats than those not exercising. [45, 46]

Over exercising can have the opposite results. Runners exceeding 60 miles per week can double their chances of becoming ill. The odds of becoming sick after a marathon are 2-5 times higher than normal, depending on the time of year. Many runners enjoy the challenge of 26.2 miles, but it is not necessary to run long distances or marathons to reap the positive effects of exercise. **Moderation is the key for the majority of those participating in an active exercise program.**

It is easier to think of adding something to your life, rather than taking something away. To begin and maintain a successful exercise program, it helps to think through what activity is appealing and reasonable, and to set realistic goals:

- Schedule a time of day. Don't worry about trying to find the perfect or exact same time every day. Flexibility is key

- Explore what types of exercise appeal most to you

- Create a mantra to help moving forward

- Find physical activities that you can enjoy

- Develop a support team or find a workout buddy

Think of exercise as something you do for the rest of your life, not just for a short period of time. Research shows that approximately 60 percent of people drop out of their exercise program after a few months. Individuals wonder why it is that after the first few weeks it becomes difficult. Taking time to analyze can set you back on course. More than likely the difficulty you are encountering is similar to other experiences – easy at first, and then challenging. Pushing through challenges results in growth.

Transition into a Program

It may be best to ease into a program – such as adding two walks on the weekend and picking which day of the week will work for the third day. After you have accomplished this for a few weeks, add a fourth day. By this time, you will begin to see the benefits of your efforts – less stress and anxiety, more restful sleep, and increased vitality. Studies show endorphins (feel-good hormones) increase with an exercise program anywhere from 4 to 12 weeks and continue for a lifetime.

An activity usually isn't a habit until you have persisted for 21 days. During the first three weeks, remind yourself of all the benefits. Reminders help, especially when the newness wears off, the cold weather hits, and it feels like sheer work. Try to push through this stage, and accept this is part of your routine. The next time you have a physical exam, your doctor and you will witness the fruits of your efforts.

Get Prepared

The night before you plan to exercise do a few things to make it easier:

- Set out your shoes, socks and clothes

- Have your bag ready with your music, towel and water if you are going to the gym

- Set the alarm with enough time to get dressed and grab a light snack before you head out the door

- If you are doing a video or DVD, have it queued up and ready to go

- Get to bed EARLY so you can feel rested, enabling you to get up the next morning

This pre-work will create a "no excuses" environment so you can be successful with your program.

Set Reasonable Expectations

Another key point is being reasonable with your expectations. It is easy to become motivated and overdo at the beginning, which can lead to injury and little or no exercise for a few weeks.

My business partner, Mitch Becker, M.D., likes to say, "The turtle wins the race," and he's right. If you start slow and plan out your steps for your new lifestyle and weight goal, your rewards will bring you to the place you desire, and you will accomplish your goals!

Focus on the reward of exercising rather than the effort it requires. I get up at 5:30 a.m. to exercise before work. Do I enjoy rising at this hour? Of course not! I would much rather wake up at 7 a.m., exercise and then go to work, but arriving at work at 11 a.m. is not an option for me. When the alarm goes off and the bed feels much better than the outside world, I ask myself, "How do you want to feel in the afternoon?" The answer is that I want to be able to concentrate and have energy. As I leave the gym, I'm already feeling better and more awake because I did get up!

You don't have to get up at 5:30 a.m. to have a successful exercise program. Making an appointment with yourself at a time you can commit to is the most important thing.

The health benefits of exercise are vast and well-documented.

A regular exercise program does the following:

- Reduces your risk of developing heart disease, high blood pressure, and adult diabetes

- Increases your immune system – e.g. less colds

- Helps with more effective stress management and decreases anxiety

- Strengthens bones and helps prevent osteoporosis

- Increases HDL cholesterol (remember the happy kind?)

- Increases your metabolism and lowers insulin resistance, which aids in losing and maintaining weight

- Increases and improves self-esteem

- Hinders the aging process by helping cells to grow and maintain health

- Increases the number of new brain cells

In March 2009, *Scientific American* reported, "Exercise and other actions may help produce extra brain cells."[47] The article stated that the exercise needs to be consistent for the additional cells to remain. These findings are analogous to exercise – if you don't use it you lose it.

For every pound of weight you lose, there is approximately 8-10 lbs less pressure or stress on the skeletal system – quite a reward for losing even a pound! Give yourself an understanding for this concept. Next time you visit the grocery store, pick up a five-pound bag of sugar, flour or potatoes and carry it while you shop. No easy feat, right?

Diabetes Prevention through Exercise

A 2002 landmark study published in the *New England Journal of Medicine* clearly demonstrated how effective lifestyle changes are in the prevention of adult-onset or Type 2 diabetes.[48] Researchers took a group of approximately 3,200 people who were at high risk of developing diabetes and divided them into three groups as follows:

Group 1 No intervention was given (the control, or placebo group)

Group 2 Put on Metformin, a diabetes drug that both prevents and treats diabetes.

Group 3 Given a change in lifestyle:
- Received guidance about exercise and nutrition

- Attended individual or group education sessions covering healthy eating and were asked to mildly decrease their caloric intake

- Exercised about 30 minutes per day, and lost about 5 percent of their body weight (about 10 pounds for a person weighing 200 pounds)

The results were striking:

- There was **no change** in the control or placebo group

- The drug group had **a 30% decrease** in the incidence of diabetes

- The lifestyle group had **a decrease of 58%** in the incidence of diabetes

This study clearly demonstrates the effectiveness of a healthy lifestyle intervening in the prevention of disease. In addition, the study published the benefits of a 30-minute walk per day coupled with minimal diet changes. This actually altered the course of the lives of the participants by preventing diabetes — a powerful payback for time invested in self-care. Think of it as compounded interest over time.

The Diabetes Prevention Study done in Finland in 2001 had an analogous protocol and achieved similar results. **Together, these studies illustrate how minor lifestyle changes like walking half an hour per day and slightly altering food consumption can have dramatic results in reducing diabetes.** This is highly positive information for those with a family history of diabetes.

Nicky's Wake-Up Call

Nicky was a young patient who got a wake-up call from her doctor about diabetes. She was 15 years old when she was referred to me by her pediatrician due to insulin resistance and risk of diabetes. She decided to take matters into her own hands and control her risk factors through diet and exercise. Here is her story:

When I stepped on the scale at my doctor's office, I am sure my face was an unpleasant mix of surprise and horror. This was not the first time my weight had jumped up in a short amount of time. However, this time the numbers went too high.

My doctor said I was on the verge of diabetes. I needed to address my situation immediately and see a nutritionist who could help me see more clearly.

I am happy to say that Susan Dopart did more than just help me see. She gave me 20/20 weight management vision.

What I learned from Susan is that the insulin I produce is not sensitive enough to elicit a normal response from my liver, fat and muscle cells. I am especially sensitive to simple carbohydrates, and foods like pasta, bread, and cereal, which had all been staples in my diet.

Exercise was another reason I was in such trouble. At one time, I worked out about eight hours a week as a competitive dancer, but injuries and personal reasons stopped me from continuing, and I did nothing to replace the exercise regimen.

After almost a year of the occasional workout and eating pasta for dinner most nights, it was a total shock to start running every day and to eat larger amounts of protein. I still have the occasional piece of pie, but even when I indulge I can feel the affect on my body. I used to get horrible stomachaches after eating loads of pasta or a baked potato, and did not know why. Now I know.

Since I've started treating my body the way it should be, there is no way I'll trade my "ignorance is bliss" way of life for what I know now. I sleep better. I'm able to run longer distances. I am losing weight, and I know I'm building the foundation for a healthier adulthood.

A one hour walk per week can prevent heart disease.

A 2001 Harvard study investigated the effects of walking in regard to cardiovascular disease in 39,000 women. The study concluded that walking one hour

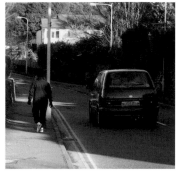

A brisk 30 minute walk cuts diabetes risk by at leat 50 percent

per week could slash cardiovascular disease in half, even in those who were overweight, had high cholesterol levels or smoked. [49]

Dr. Steven Blair, professor of Exercise Science at the University of South Carolina and former director of the Cooper Institute, states:

"Moderate levels of cardiorespiratory fitness are associated with a 50 percent lower death rate, and this applies in both women and men."

Dr. Blair defines moderate intensity exercise as walking for 30 minutes on five or more days of the week.

What about weight and exercise?

In 2008, the University of Pittsburg published a study in the *Archives of Internal Medicine*. The researchers observed obese and overweight woman over a period of three years who followed a lower calorie diet and exercised. They discovered that the women who were able to maintain a 10 percent loss of body weight over the three-year time period exercised an average of 275 minutes per week, or an average of 55 minutes five times a week. This weight loss study validated that lower calorie intake, coupled with exercise, can maintain weight loss. [50]

Similar studies have validated these results. Continuous exercise is critical to maintaining a 10 percent loss of weight over the long run. **Changing your food plan drives the weight loss, but the exercise is critical in maintaining it!**

Let's look at the basics:

What type of exercise is important? Above all, it's about finding something you enjoy. Some people dislike the gym and would rather use a video at home. There are many interesting ways to move your body – roller skating or rollerblading, ice-skating, hiking, jumping rope, dance classes (jazz, hip-hop, salsa, etc.), belly dancing, spinning, rowing, canoeing, etc. Think of something you have been tempted to investigate but never did. There are endless ways to move and enjoy being in your body. To help with longevity, it's essential to choose something you find appealing, fun and enjoyable, or at least tolerable.

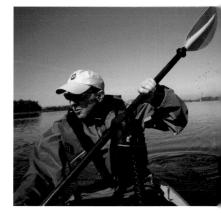

And if you need further motivation, reflect for a moment on this: What would happen if you had a health or age-related issue which prevented you from exercising? This was all too true in my own life after I had a bike accident, and it has made a difference in how I view my ability to exercise now.

I remember lying in bed after my accident wanting more than anything to be outside - take a walk, a run – anything active just to get out of my physical and emotional pain. As I write this section of the book, I now realize that one of the reasons I get up each morning and exercise is because I CAN!

There was a time in my life when I could not even walk down the hall without assistance. Lucky for me that was only a temporary state. But the lesson I learned is … take hold of the benefits of exercise now since you do not know what the future may hold.

At the beginning, exercise is often uncomfortable. Our joints are not accustomed to moving and working through some discomfort may be necessary. Discomfort is okay, but not pain. **If you are in pain, it would be prudent to see your physician before embarking on a program, just in case you have an injury or a medical issue that requires attention.** Listen to your body as you progress with your program.

Find a Plan or Routine

Find a rhythm to ensure success – something that accommodates **aerobic, strength and stretching**. Increasing your heart rate at least four times a week, whether it is going to the gym, taking a brisk walk, a bike ride, or a dance class is vital. It is essential to increase your heart rate at least three times a week to maintain your fitness level, four times a week to increase fitness and five to six times a week to build muscle and lose weight.

Start with 15-20 minutes of walking. Within hours after a walk your blood pressure and blood sugar can be in balance, mood can be lifted, and energy increased for the rest of the day. The research is illuminating – even walking 30 minutes per day will immensely help or eliminate many health issues, including weight gain.

Stepping it Up

Interval training is a type of intense cardiovascular training that is very effective in jump starting one's metabolism and increasing fat loss. It involves short bursts of speed intertwined within your cardiovascular workout. It is almost like shocking your body and pushing yourself to your limit for 20 seconds to several minutes, with a moderate intensity period of several minutes, followed by a high intensity period and a moderate period and so forth for at least 30 minutes. Check with your medical doctor before you start this type of program.

An example of interval training on an elliptical machine would entail:

- Working at a moderate level at a lower heart rate (such as 110-120 beats per minute) for 10 minutes

- Working out at a higher heart rate (such as 140-150 beats per minute) for 2-3 minutes

- Followed by a lower heart rate for 10 minutes, a higher heart rate for 2-3 minutes and so forth

Interval training once or twice a week can greatly improve fitness and weight loss. This type of exercise should only be done by someone who is in shape and needs to bring their fitness to the next level. By combining interval training with strength training you will be metabolizing fat at an even greater level. Since you are increasing your muscle mass, your metabolism will remain elevated for at least 48 hours after the workout. Doing only aerobic exercise utilizes calories during the workout and for up to 24 hours afterward, depending on the intensity of the exercise. To maximize your health and weight loss, both are needed.

It is important to be in tune with your body when you do interval training. This type of exercise is not for the novice, or those with cardiovascular problems. Be sure to check with your physician before starting an interval training program.

Resistance is the key to building muscle.

For many decades it was thought that aerobic activity was all that was needed and doing strength work was virtually ignored. Then **strength work** was re-evaluated and discovered to be important for many areas such as:

- increasing metabolism

- increasing muscle strength and tone

- preventing bone loss and osteoporosis

- lowering the risk of arthritis or lowering pain associated with arthritis

Strength training is critical, especially as you age, since your metabolism drops from bone and muscle loss. Lifting weights or doing resistance training, such as calisthenics or using bands, will maintain muscle integrity. By keeping your metabolism working at higher levels this allows your body to utilize consumed nutrients in a more efficient manner.

Different types of strength building include weights, bands, Pilates, or a yoga class incorporating strength work. Studies show strength work twice a week is essential, and if you can, three times a week is even better.

Don't forget to stretch

Stretching often is the ignored component of exercise. It may be one of the most important activities as stretching allows one to continue an

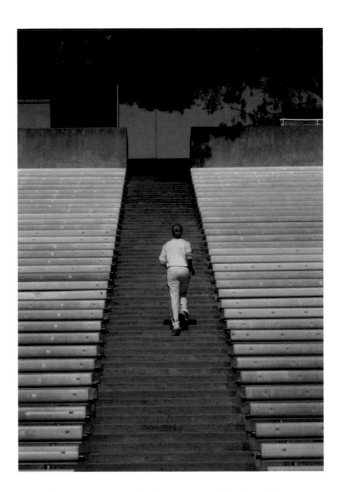

exercise program to help prevent injuries. Try to stretch every day and have longer stretch sessions at least two or three times a week.

Training

The modalities of exercise are vast. The key is finding a format you can enjoy on a long-term basis, even if the schedule is tight. If motivation is a problem, a trainer can help you get started by developing routines specifically for your needs. A trainer will also teach you how to exercise correctly to avoid injury.

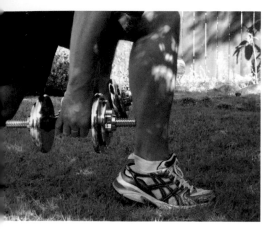

I know from personal experience that trainers can push you far beyond the limits you can push on your own and help you reach personal goals sooner. Many people have benefited from working with a trainer. If you decide to hire a trainer, inquire about the trainer's education, training, certifications and references before you begin. Inquire what modalities the trainer has planned for you and check with your physician before you begin.

The following depicts how a client was helped by combining professional help to overcome serious health problems.

Jim's Fitness Story

Jim came to see me for a nutrition consult five years ago. He was 56 years old, 5'8" and weighed 296 lbs. For most of his life he had been active in sports and was an avid snow skier. He owned a construction management firm in Los Angeles and was constantly on his feet managing and overseeing projects. Here is his story.

Over the course of 12 years I had slowly gained weight. My weight climbed from a low of 180 pounds when I was in the Army to a high of 296 pounds. I had difficulty sleeping, had orthopedic issues, was depressed and used food to calm my anxiety on a daily basis. I didn't even recognize myself in the mirror.

I developed sciatica, which is an inflammation of the sciatic nerve in the hip. The facets of my spine were impinging my spinal nerves. I couldn't sit, bend, or lay down without tremendous pain. Standing on my feet all day with the additional weight caused my feet to become inflamed. I sank into a deep depression. It was like waking up to a nightmare every day.

I was coordinating a project on a loft downtown that was four stories high. Frequently the elevator was broken, and I had to walk up and down the four flights of stairs. Due to the weight gain, I frequently had swollen feet, and suffered with back pain.

One day as I was walking up the stairs, I felt like I was having a heart attack – pain in the chest, back and shoulder. I was scared. My doctor explained that I'd had a major reaction to an anti-inflammatory drug. I had to discontinue it. Back surgery was an option, but I wanted to explore other options.

I asked my doctor to refer me to a physical therapist. Life had become so uncomfortable and miserable. I knew I had to make a change. There was no choice.

The physical therapist helped me begin to regain my mobility. She suggested I visit Susan to help with my weight. Susan showed me how to rebalance my food choices. I slowly shifted. I realized that if I wanted to have a happy and fulfilling life, I needed to change my mental outlook, eat the right foods and add exercise. I decided I would rather make these lifestyle changes than go the surgery route for my back.

Susan referred me to a private trainer. He had experience in eating disorders and structural issues. He told me that **my only goal should be to not quit.**

In about six months, I realized I enjoyed exercising! It made me feel better and kept me mentally tough, too. I went from 296 lbs. to 214 lbs. over the course of about five years.

By adding some of the principles I was learning from Susan, everything started to improve as I maintained the balance between food and exercise.

Weighing less, I developed more flexibility. My feet no longer hurt. My sciatica and nerve impingement disappeared. My stress level went down. I began sleeping well. **I also discovered that good habits created more good habits.** When I finished a hard workout, my body craved lean protein and vegetables.

The weight loss and exercise program gave me the zeal for life I had in my 20s and 30's. I changed my software, not my hardware. There is no going back! Never! The road of life will always have bumps, but good healthy food and exercise will help to smooth it out.

Incorporating exercise into your routine can restore balance to your life. Physical health coupled with mental benefits brings harmony to your system. Remember, you were built to move. Once you begin to experience the rewards, there may be no turning back! You may ask yourself, "Why didn't I do this sooner?" It does not matter when you start – what's important is that you are doing it. Keep going. Keep moving for life.

Summary

Exercise is like a magic pill! Something as easy as a half hour walk per day could be the bridge between disease and health – preventing diabetes, heart disease, arthritis, osteoporosis, improving sleep, losing and maintaining weight. There's nothing else that delivers major benefits in a short period of time.

Sleep

Have you ever wondered why as soon as you get on an airplane you feel like taking a nap? Or on vacation you sleep more deeply? Perhaps being out of our normal environments lowers our stress levels. We sleep better without the distractions of everyday life. How do we achieve this restful sleep, and why is sleep so important to our health?

Sleep is essential to weight management and appetite control. Studies show that Americans sleep 7.5 hours per night — 1.5 hours less than our grandparents slept. The *National Sleep Foundation* estimates that more than 63 percent of Americans do not get the recommended eight hours of sleep per night.

In 2002, *Science News* stated that, "The country's sleep debt may be contributing to its current epidemics of obesity, diabetes and cardiovascular disease." [51]

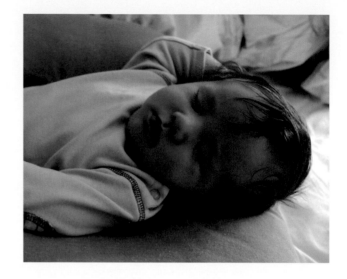

Sleep can affect:

- weight gain or loss

- hunger levels

- how well insulin works and whether diabetes develops

- the aging process

- susceptibility to colds and illness

- a person's capacity to learn new material

Sleep Studies

In 2004, researchers at Columbia University examined sleep patterns and obesity rates among those who had participated in the government's National Health and Nutrition Examination Survey from 1982-84 and then again in 1987. [52] They looked at the records of approximately 6,000 people ages 32-59 and categorized them by the amount of sleep they had per night. Normal sleepers were those who slept 7-9 hours per night.

The findings were quite astounding. Participants who slept:

- 2-4 hours per night were 73 percent more likely to be obese than the normal sleepers

- 5 hours per night were 50 percent more likely to be obese

- 6 hours per night were 23 percent more likely to be obese

- 10 or more hours per evening were 11 percent less likely to be obese

This study was an epidemiologic study, which shows association rather than cause and effect. The researchers theorized that lack of sleep may affect several hormones related to appetite and food intake, such as leptin and ghrelin (remember leptin lowers the appetite and ghrelin grows it – see *Protein chapter*).

Lack of sleep affects how HUNGRY you are during the day

Eve Van Cauter of the University of Chicago has done 25 years of research on hormones affecting sleep. In 2004, she found that sleep deprivation activates a small part of the hypothalamus (a region

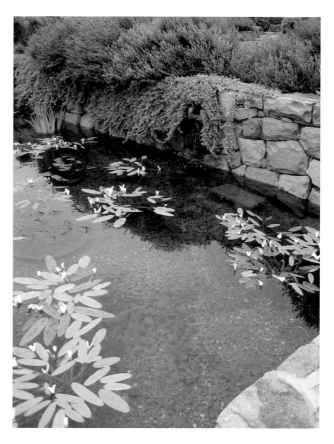

of the brain) that is involved in appetite regulation.[53] Her studies show how sleep duration has a major impact on the hormone leptin. **When people are sleep-deprived, their leptin levels are lower, which may cause the body to crave more food.**

Van Cauter and colleagues also conducted a study to see if sleep deprivation altered appetite.[54] They tested men who slept four hours for two consecutive nights followed by 10-hours' sleep for two consecutive nights. They found that after sleeping for four hours versus the 10, the men had:

- leptin levels that were 18 percent lower

- ghrelin levels that were 28 percent higher

The men said they were much hungrier than usual and craved salty, sweet food. One compounding issue: a drop in leptin can signal the body to slow down the metabolism. Sleep deprivation not only increases hunger levels, but lowers metabolism — not a good combination for weight loss.

Lack of sleep can affect how well your insulin functions and whether you get diabetes.

An earlier study done by Van Cauter in 1999 at the University of Chicago tracked how lack of sleep in men affects the body and how the body handles food. [55] The study looked at young men who slept four hours per night for six nights. The findings showed that the men's blood sugars or glucose levels spiked higher after breakfast than when they slept for nine hours per night. The study revealed the men's insulin levels had 40 percent lower sensitivity when they were sleep deprived than when they slept for the longer period of time.

Researcher James Gangwisch of Columbia University reported in 2007 that people who get less than five hours of sleep per night are significantly more likely to have Type 2 diabetes. [56]

Three large studies published in *Nature Genetics* in December 2008 describe the first genetic link between sleep and Type 2 diabetes. These studies link two trends in the U.S. – rising diabetes rates and falling sleep trends, or generally lack of sleep.

Getting a cold? Want to look good? Get some sleep!

In 2009, Sheldon Cohen and colleagues at Carnegie Mellon University studied how sleep habits can increase susceptibility to colds.[57] They found people who slept less than seven hours a night were three times more likely to catch a cold than those who sleep eight hours or more per night. The researchers concluded that sleep disruption interferes with the immune system's ability to regulate itself.

Another finding from Van Cauter's 1999 study about sleep and food revealed a correlation between sleep and aging. On the days the men had sleep deprivation, they showed higher levels of cortisol (see *Stress chapter*). "Differences also showed up in the men's nervous systems and thyroid hormone concentrations that made them look, on lab tests, decades older than they actually were – potentially paving the way for high blood pressure and other conditions more common with age." The bottom line? **Sleeping can make a difference in looking youthful or aged.**

Sleep Resets Your Brain

Chiara Cirelli of the University of Wisconsin-Madison and her colleagues conduct ongoing research on why sleep is necessary. They have found that sleep changes and resets the brain to be able to continue learning new things. It is as if sleep pushes the reset button on your brain. Key point: **sleep is essential to all the systems within our body.**

Gender Differences

Women who don't get enough restful sleep are more likely to be moody, upset, or unwell. Men have about 15-20 times more testosterone than women. Without enough sleep, they can function well enough throughout the day. Without sleep, women do not function as well on many levels and lack vitality and a sense of well-being.

Summary

Some of us may be diligent about balancing our diets, eating when hungry, stopping when we are satisfied and maintaining regular exercise. However, others of us may not lose weight until we are able to obtain adequate rest.

Great health begins with a good night's sleep. Sleep **resets** the systems in your body to:

- Keep your appetite normal

- Help your insulin work efficiently

- Assist your body with maintaining a normal weight

- Keep you healthy

- Learn new material

Without sleep, the rest of the systems of our bodies do not function the way they were intended. So, keep rest and slumber a priority!

Stress

"Stress" is a catch-all term we hear or see each day. TV infomercials, pharmacies, billboards, and printed ads all promote stress relief pills or products you can purchase to help calm or lower or control your stress. If only the claims for special music, lavender pillows or pills could permanently alter stress! But they can't.

Stress is a part of being human and therefore is a major influence affecting our health and weight. In fact, many experts claim stress alters virtually every chemical function in our body. Stress can:

- Influence whether you store or lose fat

- Increase blood sugars and the possibility of becoming diabetic

- Increase cholesterol levels and the risk of heart disease

- Lower the immune system and increase a person's chances of getting a cold or the flu

- Affect sleep patterns

Stress and the Adrenal System

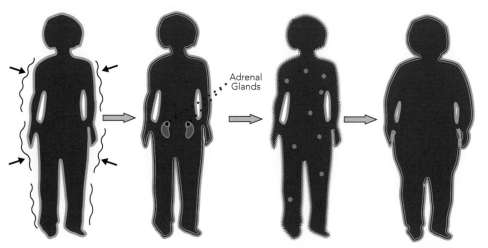

Adrenal Glands

If cortisol remains elevated for long periods of time there is:

- increase in fat storage

- increased cholesterol levels

- increased blood sugars

- decreased immune function

outside stress causes a chain reaction in the body

when stressed, the adrenals release the hormone cortisol

cortisol is released throughout the body during this "flight or fight" response

effects of cortisol remaining elevated

When our bodies are stressed, the adrenals release a hormone called cortisol. Cortisol is released during the "flight or fight response," which is the adapted response we instantly employ when under attack or in preparation for conflict.

Having cortisol levels that are elevated for prolonged periods of time can change our internal chemistry since the adrenal glands are linked to almost every endocrine gland in the body. Our immunity decreases, blood sugars increase, and cholesterol levels go up. High levels of cortisol can accelerate fat storage, especially around the mid section. Many people with high cortisol levels crave high-fat, high-sugar foods and this exacerbates the cycle.

Stress and Your Metabolism

In 1993, Per Bjorntorp, a researcher in Sweden at the University of Goteborg, coined the phrase "Civilization Syndrome," to describe how stress may be a major source of risk for metabolic abnormalities leading to chronic disease [58]

Translation: Stress can change your metabolism in significant ways to increase disease in your body.

In addition, Bjorntorp reported that if the stress is chronic and coupled with high amounts of alcohol, overeating and/or smoking, it can lead to a change in your nervous or endocrine system. This is significant because the endocrine system controls virtually every cell, organ, or function in your body, including the thyroid, adrenal glands, reproductive glands, and metabolism.

An elevated endocrine response leads to visceral (deep tissue in the mid section) obesity, insulin resistance, high blood pressure, high cholesterol, adult diabetes, and cardiovascular disease. It's safe to say that stress and overindulgences cause major health issues.

Telomeres and Aging

In 2008, we heard about the connection between stress and *telomeres* – DNA complexes on the ends of chromosomes. Researcher Elizabeth Blackburn compares telomeres to the tips at the ends of new shoelaces which prevent unraveling.

Chronic stress has been linked to aging and increased signs of aging. A 2004 study at the University of California at San Francisco investigated healthy women between the ages of 20 and 50 who were the primary caregivers for their children [59] Sixty-seven percent of the women were the primary caregiver for a chronically sick child.

The researchers measured the length of telomeres in these women and discovered a striking connection between stress and telomere length. Mothers with increased stress levels had significantly shorter telomeres than the women who reported lower stress levels. The women with higher stressors had telomeres resembling women 10 years older.

As you age, your telomeres shorten.

As related to these findings, Blackburn wrote, "This is the first evidence that chronic psychological stress – and how a person perceives that stress – may damp down telomerase and have significant impact on the length of telomeres, suggesting that stress may modulate cellular aging."

Studies done since this time have shown a connection between telomere length and aging, but have not been conclusive with a direct correlation. However, research still points to the fact that stress has a major impact on all the cells of the body, which in turn can affect the way our bodies process food.

Does exercise affect telomeres?

In 2008, researchers at the University of Maryland studied the effects of varying levels of exercise affecting length of telomeres.[60]   The results showed that moderate physical activity provided a protective effect on telomere length compared to low or high levels of exercise.

Even when we are stressed, moderate exercise provides a protective effect on telomeres.

So what does this tell us?

Stress can keep our bodies stuck when attempting to lose weight and restore health and balance. I've see this first hand. Many of my clients ate well and exercised, but did not lose weight due to high levels of stress. As they learned to manage stress with various modalities, they were able to lose weight.

Changing our eating habits can help the body reverse these metabolic responses due to stress, especially when coupled with moderate exercise.

Exercise lowers cortisol levels in your body. Working out not only lowers cortisol levels, but increases endorphins, which in turn, dynamically decreases stress levels.

Simplifying Stress

Stress is always going to be a part of our lives. A major defense against the impact of stress is to equip yourself with elements to buffer and handle stress. A balanced diet and moderate exercise are easy steps to take to help handle stress.

In addition to exercise, meditation and yoga can help to lower stress and aid in weight loss.   Restful sleep on a regular basis is crucial for assisting the adrenal system to function and for lowering stress levels. Becoming aware of how stress affects your life can start the process of change.

Nurture yourself by taking small breaks. Step away from work during the course of your day. Breathe deeply, exhale longer. Relax. Stretch. Repeat. Enjoy nature. Be well.

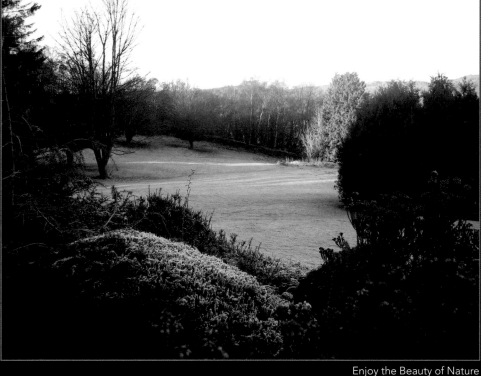
Enjoy the Beauty of Nature

Family History and Life Stages

Family Weight History

When looking at your health and weight, consider your family history. What does your family look like? This includes your mother, father, siblings, aunts, uncles, grandparents, and cousins. If you came from an overweight family, the probability of a weight issue is more likely than if you came from a thin family.

I still remember the days in college when I went to aerobics. There were two sisters who usually stood in front of me – tall, thin, and with figures most women would die for. They had exactly the same body type and you could not tell them apart from the back, except for their hair color. This demonstrated to me early on how genetics can influence body types and shapes.

However, your family history need not be your destiny. Coming from an overweight family does not mean you are destined to a lifetime of weight issues – it just means you may have to be more diligent balancing your diet, watching your bites and having consistent exercise as part of your overall routine.

My family ancestry consists of overweight Italian women. Becoming a registered dietitian was my quest for not succumbing to that plight. I am not a naturally thin person. I have to consciously watch all my bites of food, exercise consistently, and maintain good self-care or my weight will quickly balloon.

If you are open to adjusting your diet, exercise patterns, and healing your relationship with food, *change is in your future*. You may not be the thinnest person on the face of the planet, but altering your lifestyle choices will keep you fit and healthy.

The Start of Genetics - Fertility and Pregnancy

Often during pregnancy people read about the importance of consuming carbohydrates and grains. In my practice many pregnant women come in for a nutrition consult. They are eating large bowls of pasta, rice, potatoes and cereal and wonder why they have gained so much weight. To complicate matters, some develop problems such as gestational diabetes and/or high blood pressure (known as *preeclampsia*) during pregnancy. Let's investigate what happens to the body during pregnancy.

Pregnancy is a state of insulin resistance. Therefore, eating a balanced diet of healthy forms of carbohydrate, protein, and good fat becomes all the more essential. Pregnant women generally need 300 more calories per day, which in no way is a license to eat for two. It is important to be in a nutritionally balanced state when thinking about becoming pregnant and at the beginning of a pregnancy.

Daily Guidelines for Pregnancy and Lactation

Here is a checklist for healthy eating for fertility, pregnancy, or breast-feeding. You'll also find some specific recommendations in the next section.

☑ **Strive for balance in your diet**
- *Protein* - lean sources of beef, lamb, chicken, and fish; eggs, nuts/seeds, nut butters at each meal and snack

- *Carbohydrates* - fruits, vegetables, and unprocessed whole grains

- *Fats* – omega-3 rich and monounsaturated fats (avocados, nuts/seeds and olive oil) on a daily basis:

  - *ALA* – found in ground flax seed

  - *DHA* -found in fish and fish oil

  - *EPA* – found in fish and fish oil

☑ **Eat or drink dairy** - 3-4 servings of organic plain low-fat cheese, cottage/ricotta cheese, milk, hard cheeses (grass-fed if possible)

☑ **Consume fruits** - 3 to 4 servings per day, including one citrus or vitamin-C rich fruit

☑ **Eat your vegetables** - dark green leafy and orange/yellow/red daily

☑ **Choose real, whole foods** - avoid processed and refined foods. Choose fresh, unprocessed foods, and as much as possible, organic and non-GMO foods and animal products that are grass fed

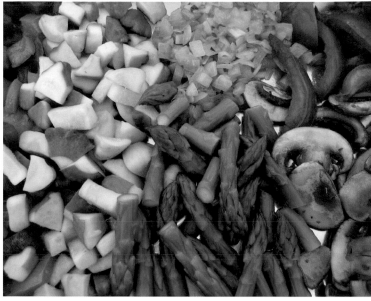

Eat the colors!

☑ Avoid diet foods or foods with non-nutritive sweeteners

☑ Minimize caffeine and **avoid alcohol**

Additional Recommendations for Mothers and Mothers-to-Be

- Include **high-quality protein** in your diet. To get the highest quality protein and maintain balanced blood sugars throughout the day, begin the day with eggs for breakfast. If you are not an egg fan, then cottage or ricotta cheese or plain yogurt mixed with fruit and nuts and seeds will provide sufficient protein, with a balance of healthy fat and carbohydrate (*see Balancing your Meals chapter for additional choices*).

- **Avoids bowls of cereal** with fruit and

milk which can lead to an increased insulin level and result in a drop in blood sugars. The blood sugar drop can create increased hunger levels and carbohydrate cravings throughout the day.

- **Have protein at lunch and dinner**, balanced with fruits, vegetables, and healthy fats such as avocado, nuts/seeds.

- **Good sources of calcium** are important such as plain yogurt, ricotta cheese, hard cheeses and milk.

- **One or two dark green leafy vegetables** such as broccoli, Brussels sprouts, spinach are important to include.

- **Include one yellow or orange vegetable** such as carrots, butternut squash, or sweet potatoes/yams.

- **Omega-3 fats are critical**. DHA *(see Fat chapter)* is important for development of the baby's brain. It may be difficult to obtain enough DHA via the diet. When breastfeeding, DHA is very important to supplement for the mood of the mother and the baby's health and well-being. Low DHA levels are linked to depression in breastfeeding mothers. Therefore, fish oil or fish oil capsules are usually necessary.

Exercise

Exercise during pregnancy is safe and can help prevent complications such as gestational diabetes and preeclampsia. Currently, only 15.1 percent of pregnant women exercise, since it is perceived as risky. [61] However, multiple research studies show exercise in early pregnancy can reduce risks of complications, improve sleep, and reduce anxiety.

Exercise has also been linked to an easier labor and delivery.

I had the privilege of hearing James Clapp, M.D., author of *Exercising Through Your Pregnancy (2002)*, at a sports nutrition conference. He is a medical research expert in prenatal exercise as well as a professor at Case Western Reserve University and at the University of Vermont College of Medicine.

He has done extensive research on how exercise lowers complications from pregnancy and improves outcomes. His research shows that regular weight bearing exercise during pregnancy lowers markers of insulin resistance and blood glucose concentration during and immediately after exercise. [62]

A 2008 study by Dr. Clapp showed that women who voluntarily maintain their exercise regimen during pregnancy continue to exercise over time at a higher level than those who stop. They also reap benefits following their pregnancies such as:

- Gaining less weight in the future (7.5 pounds versus 22 pounds)

- Deposit less fat (4.8 pounds versus 14.7 pounds)

- Have increased fitness

- Have a lower risk of cardiovascular disease even during the peri-menopausal period. [63]

If you are a high-risk pregnancy, exercise may not be an option. It is always best to get your doctor's approval for the type and modality of exercise that is safe for you and your baby.

Respect for your baby's health and your health begins prior to getting pregnant. Begin your pregnancy with a balanced eating and exercise program, and maintain that balance throughout your pregnancy. I suggest meeting with a registered dietitian prior to getting pregnant, or soon after you discover you are pregnant. A registered dietitian can create an individualized plan that takes into account your particular genetics and family history.

During the 2009 American Diabetes Association postgraduate session I attended in New York, researchers stated how a woman's diet influences the weight and body fat of her child in utero. Therefore, having a healthy diet during pregnancy has the potential to greatly influence future generations.

Avoiding the Menopausal Middle

A large group of patients who commonly come in for weight management are perimenopausal and postmenopausal women. Weight gain during this time is common for a variety of reasons. Many women who have not had weight issues throughout their lives suddenly find themselves gaining weight. Those who have had weight issues find this issue compounded exponentially. Coupling this change with the other physiological changes of menopause creates a difficult time for many women.

One key to this season in life is linked to hormones. Hormones are basically messengers that give the body signals about what to do, similar to traffic lights. Hormones can control the immune system, metabolism, and reproduction, in addition to many other systems in the body. During menopause these systems can change or become disrupted.

Elizabeth Lee Vliet, M.D., a medical expert in women's health and author of *Women, Weight and*

Hormones: A Weight Loss Plan for Women Over 35, recommends women check their hormone levels to establish a baseline and then work with a reliable physician to regulate them. [64] Among some of the tests she recommends are fasting insulin levels, thyroid hormones, ovarian hormones (estradiol, progesterone, testosterone), cortisol, cholesterol panel, and CBC.

Laboratory tests to consider during perimenopause and menopause include:

- FSH
- Estrogen
- Progesterone
- Testosterone
- Insulin
- Cortisol
- DHEA-sulfate
- TSH, free T3, free T4 (thyroid levels)

Discuss with your personal physician what the options are for your situation and genetics.

A balanced diet and lifestyle is critical:

- Regular balanced meals with high-quality protein
- Fruits, vegetables and healthy carbohydrate sources at meals and snacks

- Healthy fats – from monounsaturated and omega-3 rich sources

- Exercise program incorporating cardiovascular and strength training

Since bone loss occurs with changes in hormones and age, weight gain around the middle is common. Weight training can stop muscle atrophy or bone losses, which will then increase the metabolic rate and stop or minimize weight gain.

In addition, exercise can assist with mood stabilization, reduction of hot flashes, anxiety and insomnia. Yoga is extremely helpful with moods and symptoms of menopause. Acupuncture also helps rebalance the systems of the body.

Is There a Male Menopause?

Research on menopause focuses mostly on females and the changes they incur as they age. However, men also experience physical changes. The most frequent disorder of sex hormones in men is called *hypogonadism*, which is usually associated with a testosterone level of less than 300 ng/dl.

Hypogonadism is linked with an increased accumulation of visceral fat *(see Diet, Disease and Medical Issues chapter),* insulin resistance and a risk of adult onset diabetes. Overweight or obese men tend to have lower testosterone levels, which may need treatment.

Men with adult onset diabetes have a 70 percent higher risk of hypogonadism.[65] A balanced diet and exercise program as described above become of utmost importance to lower visceral fat and restore balance in the body. In addition, testosterone levels need to be monitored and if low, supplemental testosterone is often prescribed by a physician.

It's important to realize that men and women share the journey of change. Mutual understanding and acceptance of the physical and emotional changes that occur over the course of our lives is essential for harmony between the sexes.

Summary

We were given our genetic makeup in utero. What we do with those genes is our choice. Since life is full of changes and ups and downs, maintaining or restoring balance becomes more important at each turn in our journey — whether it is pregnancy, mid-life or later in life.

"If your lifestyle does not control your body—eventually your body will control your lifestyle...the choice is yours!"

— Ern Baxter, author of I Almost Died

Diet, Disease and Medical Issues

There are many medical issues that can be brought on by weight gain, unbalanced eating or an unhealthy lifestyle. However, some medical issues are purely genetic and may not respond to diet or exercise. Sorting out how to discern which are inherently genetic and those that are self-imposed can be challenging. Additionally, some issues may be a combination of genetics and lifestyle.

In this chapter, we'll look at the connection between diet and disease and focus on some common conditions – diabetes, PCOS, cancer, hypertension and heart disease, osteoporosis, arthritis and GERD. Although each has its own set of medical challenges, I believe that diet and lifestyle can influence treatment for the better.

Connecting Diet and Disease

Time and time again studies done by prominent researchers continue to show the correlation between diet and disease. Researchers have found direct associations among food, exercise, stress, sleep, weight and health. It's clear that lifestyle impacts vitality and the aging process more than we previously thought. Currently, one in three Americans is overweight, and the numbers are rapidly rising. It is expected that more than 50 percent of the American population will be overweight by the year 2030.

The Nurses' Health Study (ongoing since 1976) and other major studies that look at health issues and risks, continue to show the relationship between increased weight and the risk of heart disease, high blood pressure, diabetes and death. Men and women gaining anywhere from 11-20 pounds were up to three times more likely to develop health issues.

A current popular topic for research is **inflammation**. We all know what happens when you sprain your ankle or hurt some part of your body – it becomes inflamed and swollen. But, there are also things going on inside the body that the naked eye can't see. That's similar to what happens when you eat something unhealthy.

What happens *internally* when you eat something harmful?

Most think nothing happens, which may be true in some instances. However, even one fast food meal can cause inflammation. For example, if you ate a fast-food hamburger, fries and a coke, here's what would happen:

1. Insulin levels rise to accommodate high glucose levels

2. Levels of trans fat in your blood can trigger free radicals or oxygenation (i.e. rust on an old car), and constriction in your blood vessels

Fast food meal with insulin level spiking and constriction of blood vessels

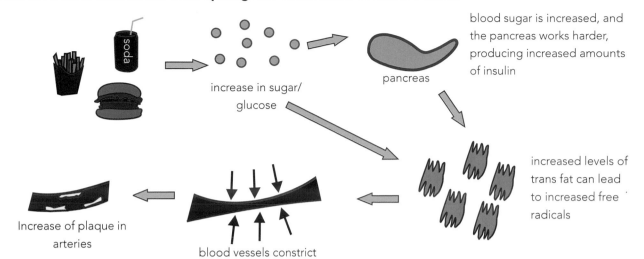

increase in sugar/ glucose

pancreas

blood sugar is increased, and the pancreas works harder, producing increased amounts of insulin

increased levels of trans fat can lead to increased free radicals

blood vessels constrict

Increase of plaque in arteries

These changes are short lived and can be turned around with a healthy meal, but what happens if you consume these foods meal after meal?

Inflammation is manifested in many forms, and triggers many health issues such as:

- high blood pressure
- heart disease
- fatty liver
- diabetes
- cancer
- gastrointestinal reflux (GERD)

One blood test used to measure inflammation in the body is called **C-reactive protein**. This measures when inflammation is high, like when the body is experiencing infection and stress, but can also be elevated due to obesity, cardiovascular disease, or diabetes. A measure greater than 3 puts someone in a higher risk category than having levels below 3.

Before diving into medical issues, let's examine the difference between visceral versus subcutaneous fat in the body since visceral fat is one of the main causes of inflammation.

Fat in the Body

Different types of dietary fat exist, but have you ever thought about fat contained within the body? There are two types of fat: *visceral* and *subcutaneous*. Subcutaneous fat is the padding beneath your skin and is not a health risk unless excessive. Think of it like the insulation in the walls of your home. **Visceral fat** is the fat that accumulates in and around the abdominal region, and is referred to as belly fat, or having a "beer belly."

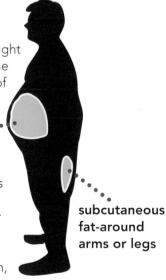

visceral/ belly fat

subcutaneous fat-around arms or legs

Visceral fat is dangerous due to the inflammatory hormones it secretes. Many people know belly fat is not attractive, but do not realize it is metabolically active tissue with blood vessels running throughout that can be dangerous or even deadly. A 1998 study published in the *Journal of Clinical Endocrinology & Metabolism* examined what happens when visceral and subcutaneous fat are observed in a Petri dish.[66] The visceral fat released three times more toxic inflammatory chemicals than the subcutaneous fat.

Visceral fat is dangerous for a variety of reasons:

- It has a direct route to the liver and can negatively increase liver function tests such as cholesterol

- It is linked with dumping inflammatory hormones into your body, which can affect your heart, kidney, and brain

- It is associated with insulin resistance, which is an inability of your body to respond appropriately to your own insulin, which in turn increases fat storage and blood sugars

- It is connected with increased rates of cancer and cancer-like growths in the body

Men with a waist circumference larger than 40 inches, or women with a 35-inch waist or greater, are at a high risk of disease due to increased visceral fat.

To measure your waist, place the tape measurement around the circumference of your waist at the point of your belly button. This measure is more important than the number on the scale: **waist size is more important than weight.**

It is important to remember that visceral fat did not come on overnight, and will not come off easily. This type of fat is stubborn. Consistency with a healthy balanced diet and exercise program is required if you want to see permanent body and health changes.

Diabetes

Diabetes is a complex metabolic endocrine disorder affecting many systems in the body. **Diabetes is considered a state of low level inflammation**. [67]

Many individuals think diabetes is caused by eating too much sugar or carbohydrates. Although consuming more carbohydrates may play a role as to whether someone is diagnosed with diabetes, it is not the main cause. Insulin resistance can be the start of diabetes *(see Carbohydrate chapter)*, but what causes insulin resistance?

The leptin/diabetes connection?

Leptin may be one of the keys to whether someone develops diabetes or not. In 2005, researchers at the University of Michigan Medical School led by Martin Myers, M.D., did a study suggesting that the hormone leptin regulates blood sugar through two different pathways – one that controls blood sugars levels via the action of insulin and another that controls appetite and fat storage. [68]

Leptin does a lot to control whether you are hungry, gain weight or get diabetes. What do the studies show?

Diabetes Study 1
In 2005, researchers at the University of Michigan Medical School took two groups of mice and genetically modified one group. [69]

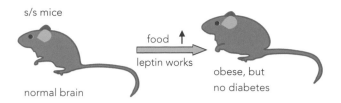

s/s mice

normal brain

food ↑
leptin works

obese, but
no diabetes

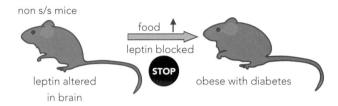

non s/s mice

food ↑
leptin blocked

STOP

leptin altered
in brain

obese with diabetes

Group 1: Called the s/s mice, they were not genetically modified, and had leptin receptors in their brains that worked normally. Although this group consumed a lot of food and became obese, they did not develop diabetes.

Group 2: Called the non s/s mice, these were genetically modified to make no leptin, and had no leptin receptors in their brain. They became obese and died of diabetes.

How does this study help us understand how to avoid becoming diabetic, even with a family history of diabetes?

Leptin has a critical role in hunger, weight and insulin regulation as it:

- is produced by the fat cells

- regulates whether you are hungry or not

- regulates energy and whether to use it for repairing your cells or storing it as fat

- is involved in the action of insulin

Therefore, if your body becomes insensitive to leptin, and in fact, develops a *leptin resistance*, the brain will signal your body that it needs more food, and your body will continue to store fat.

As part of a study on leptin, Judith Altarejos, Ph.D., of the Salk Research Institute, wrote that, "**Obesity results when the brain becomes 'deaf' to the leptin signals.**"

If you consume a high-carbohydrate diet composed of starchy and processed foods, your pancreas releases increased amounts of insulin to try to use the sugar or store it as fat in order to move it out of the blood stream. This process can start slowly, and if your diet does not change, you will continue to gain weight. The insulin-producing cells of your pancreas, known as the beta cells, can slowly start to die during this process.

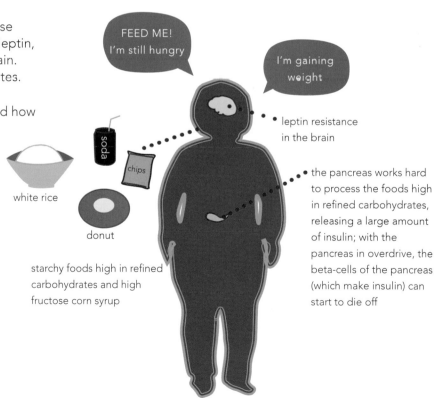

FEED ME!
I'm still hungry

I'm gaining weight

leptin resistance in the brain

the pancreas works hard to process the foods high in refined carbohydrates, releasing a large amount of insulin; with the pancreas in overdrive, the beta-cells of the pancreas (which make insulin) can start to die off

white rice

soda

chips

donut

starchy foods high in refined carbohydrates and high fructose corn syrup

In addition, your brain can develop a leptin resistance. The combination of the leptin resistance in the brain and the pancreas working hard to keep your blood sugar normal can lead to both weight gain and diabetes.

The more insulin the pancreas continues to pump out, the more insulin resistant the body becomes. It is almost like trying to pump gas into your car, but the car won't accept the gas or use it properly.

As the body becomes more insulin resistant, it becomes increasingly more leptin resistant, making weight loss very difficult. Can we turn this viscous cycle around? Let's look at another study which revealed the relationship between fructose consumption and leptin resistance before we answer this question.

Diabetes Study 2

In 2008, researchers at the University of Florida College of Medicine looked at whether high levels of fructose from high-sugar foods (which are half fructose) and foods with high fructose corn syrup could change the way leptin works in the body. [70]

Two groups of rats were fed similar diets, but one group was fed 60 percent fructose (from sugar and foods containing high fructose corn syrup) and the other received a low fructose diet, meaning they were fed their regular diets without additional high fructose or high sugar foods. This study is not talking about natural fructose containing foods like fruit, but foods sweetened with high fructose corn syrup or processed foods with sugar.

The researchers discovered that the rats fed a high fructose diet for six months had higher levels of triglycerides, which hindered the brain's response to leptin. If leptin does not reach the brain, the brain will not send out the signal to stop eating.

After six months, both groups of rats were fed

a high fat diet for two weeks, similar to a typical American diet. The rats fed the high fructose diet ate more food during the two weeks than the low fructose rat group, and rapidly gained weight (more than the low fructose group).

These researchers concluded that eating a high fructose diet increased triglycerides. High triglycerides change the way leptin works in the brain, blocking the signal to stop eating.

Translation: Eating processed high sugar foods or foods sweetened with high fructose corn syrup can change your metabolism and make you hungry.

Leptin could be compared to a valve that shuts off hunger.

Basically, our typical American diet with high fructose, high starchy, high fat foods can trigger this leptin resistance and cause a host of problems. How do we reverse weight gain and diabetes?

Reversing Leptin Resistance

Surender Arora, M.D., an endocrinologist and researcher at Kings Hospital in New York, summarizes causes of inflammation related to the diet:

"Excess intake of processed carbohydrates sets up a vicious cycle whereby the transient spikes in blood glucose and insulin early after a meal trigger reactive hypoglycemia and hunger. The chronic consumption of a diet high in processed carbohydrates leads to visceral fat, which increases insulin resistance and inflammation and predisposes one to diabetes, hypertension, and cardiovascular disease. In contrast, restriction of refined carbohydrates will

improve the post-prandial (after meals) levels of both glucose and triglycerides levels and can reduce intra-abdominal fat, particularly in individuals with insulin resistance." [71,72]

Lowering your intake of refined and processed carbohydrates and increasing protein and healthy fats such as omega-3's and monounsaturated can open the shut-off valve, helping you feel satisfied and in control of your food. If you change your diet by eating healthy carbohydrates such as fruits and vegetables (and avoid processed or refined carbohydrates) you will have normal blood sugars and possibly avoid getting insulin resistance, diabetes, high blood pressure or heart disease.

Translation: Normal blood sugars will lower your triglycerides, which can lower the leptin resistance in the brain, help you feel full, lower your level of insulin resistance and decrease your weight.

The **balance** of your diet becomes critical in controlling this metabolic problem. **Calories in are not equal to calories out**. Anssi H. Manninen, Ph.D., at the University of Oulu in Finland has done extensive research on whether this common expression is true. In his 2004 paper, *Is a calorie really a calorie? Metabolic advantage of low carbohydrate diets*, published in the *Journal of International Society of Sports Nutrition*, he discusses how different diets lead to different biochemical pathways that are not equivalent when correctly compared through the laws of thermodynamics. [73]

Furthermore, a high carbohydrate low fat diet is unsatisfactory for overweight individuals. **Whether the issue is leptin or insulin signaling, sufficient studies exist to show that moderating your intake of carbohydrate can significantly lower insulin resistance, which in turn can have an enormous effect on whether someone develops diabetes.**

How can you check if you are at risk for diabetes?

Each year I attend the American Diabetes Association (ADA) postgraduate courses, which provide the most up-to-date information on diabetes diagnosis and treatment. The ADA recommends you monitor your blood levels using the parameters below to determine if you are at risk for diabetes.

Monitor Your Levels
Don't rely on how you feel, since pre-diabetes can be silent in the body until your blood sugars are dangerously elevated. Have a physical once a year and ask your physician to monitor:

- insulin
- c-peptide
- glycosylated hemoglobin A1C

Your fasting insulin levels should be less than 10 and your c-peptide should be less than 4.5, depending on the lab's norms. The c-peptide and insulin measure how hard your pancreas is working to keep your blood sugars normal.

The glycosylated hemoglobin A1C measures what your blood sugar has been averaging over the previous three months. Normal levels are between 4 and 6.5. These tests are outside of the normal blood work checked, so you may need to ask your physician to add them.

An easy way to see if you are pre-diabetic is to look at what your fasting glucose level is over time. Pre-diabetes has been linked to a fasting glucose level of over 95. A fasting glucose in the 95-115 range could indicate pre-diabetes or diabetes. Keeping copies of your blood work over the years helps you compare your levels.

Regulation of blood sugars is critical since it can lead to a host of other medical issues. Large increases in blood sugar are associated with high blood pressure, blood clot formations, and decreased blood flow to the tissues of the heart. In addition, if blood sugars stay elevated, it leads to high insulin levels, which have been linked to an increased risk of cancer.

Caffeine: A Connection to Diabetes?

Recent studies link caffeine to higher blood sugars. James Lane, Ph.D., a researcher at Duke University, has done a vast amount of research on caffeine and diabetes. His most recent study in 2008 found that when subjects drank four cups of coffee their blood sugars increased by eight percent. [74] Another researcher who has worked alongside Dr. Lane, Richard Surwit, M.D., wrote a book called *The Mind-Body Diabetes Revolution*. Dr. Surwit, a professor of medical psychology at Duke University Medical Center, discusses his years of findings working with diabetics and how caffeine increases blood sugars. He states:

> "Caffeine increases levels of the stress hormone epinephrine* and also makes us more responsive to the epinephrine circulating in the bloodstream. As a result, your heart beats faster, your blood pressure increases, blood sugars rise and you feel an initial jolt of energy. However, this jolt puts your body in fight-or-flight mode….in short, caffeine makes you particularly sensitive to stress." [75]

Dr. Surwit reports that **caffeine increases insulin levels by 42 percent and decreases insulin sensitivity by 25 percent.** He advises those with diabetes to limit their intake of caffeine. Surwit also proposes that people with diabetes have systems that are more susceptible to the physiological effects of stress than those without diabetes, and caffeine can exacerbate stress.

Pre-diabetes and diabetes respond very well to lifestyle changes. In a world where we have so much information at our fingertips, it is still a wonder that diabetes is vastly rampant and increasing. With a balanced diet and some daily activity, diabetes could be put to rest in many individuals *(see Exercise chapter)*.

Including protein at each meal with moderate amounts of carbohydrate in the form of fruits, vegetables, nuts, seeds, and a balance of monounsaturated and omega-3 rich fats may significantly help with avoiding diabetes. Of course stress, exercise and sleep also play an important role and need to be addressed at an individual level. The chemical structure of caffeine in tea has less of an effect on the body than caffeine in coffee. If you are at risk for diabetes or have diabetes, it might be worth switching to tea since it has a much gentler effect on the system, besides having beneficial qualities to your body *(see Phytochemical chapter)*.

Nuts — Not just for squirrels

Epidemiological (cause and effect) studies consistently indicate that consumption of nuts at least five times a week will reduce diabetes and heart disease risks by 20-50 percent. Replacing carbohydrates with monounsaturated fats (i.e. nuts and olive oil) lowers the blood sugars, which

*Epinephrine is a hormone and neurotransmitter that is involved in the "flight or flight" response. When your body is in a stressful situation, epinephrine is released into your system. Most people think of epinephrine as the lay word adrenalin.

in turn lower oxidative stress in the body and inflammation.[76]   So, enjoy raw or dry roasted nuts and know you are treating your body very well indeed!

Gestational Diabetes

Since pregnancy is a state of insulin resistance, many women are susceptible to blood sugar changes. Women with gestational diabetes (diabetes brought on by hormones in pregnancy) have a high propensity to have diabetes later in life. *Gestational diabetes mellitus* is defined as carbohydrate intolerance of variable severity with onset of first recognition during pregnancy.[77]

Having gestational diabetes can almost be looked at as a blessing since it is a forewarning and can be treated. If women with gestational diabetes change their diets and lifestyle both during pregnancy and afterward, they can avoid getting adult onset or Type 2 diabetes in the future. Of course, this is not always the case, but a diet and exercise alteration now can deter or obliterate diabetes later in life for many women.

Baby boomers may have been insulin resistant or developed gestational diabetes without knowing it due to a lack of refined early testing procedures that are now done with current practices. If you gained over 50 pounds when you were pregnant, there is a good chance you might fall into this category. If that's the case, it would be wise to have your physician monitor your blood levels, including insulin, c-peptide and glycosylated hemoglobin A1C.

Polycystic Ovarian Syndrome (PCOS)

There is a spectrum of menstrual disorders which exist, but the prevalent one is Polycystic Ovarian Syndrome. Polycystic Ovarian Syndrome (PCOS) is an endocrine disorder affecting about 6-10 percent of women who are of reproductive age.[78] PCOS is hard to diagnose and therefore missed by health care professionals. If a woman has less than eight menstrual cycles per year, there is an 80 percent chance she runs the risk of having PCOS.

Although 10 percent of women with PCOS are lean with no weight issues, 90 percent have insulin resistance and problematic weight issues. PCOS is diagnosed by three main features: [79]

1. Hyperandrogenism (high levels of male hormones, such as testosterone)

2. Anovulation (lack of ovulation)

3. Polycystic ovaries

Common diagnostic laboratory measures include, but are not limited to:

- c-peptide (measures insulin output by the pancreas)

- glycosylated hemoglobin A1C (measures the previous three-month blood sugar average)

- fasting glucose level (levels above 100 can be indicative of insulin resistance)

- fasting insulin (levels above 10 can be indicative of insulin resistance)

- oral glucose tolerance test

- total and free testosterone

- DHEA-sulfate

- FSH (follicle stimulating hormone)

- LH (luteinizing hormone)

- cholesterol panel (total, HDL, LDL, triglycerides)

- c-reactive protein (measures inflammation in the body)

Abnormalities in laboratory blood work we see in women with PCOS are:

- fasting glucose levels above 100

- glycosylated hemoglobin A1C above 5.5

- high triglyceride levels

- high LDL (remember the lousy) cholesterol

- low HDL (happy) cholesterol

Other signs and symptoms of having PCOS are:

- hair growth on the face or body called *hirsutism*

- acne or oily skin

- depression or mood swings

- frequent miscarriages

- infertility

Women with PCOS have a two-fold risk of myocardial infarction (heart attack), equal to a woman of 70 years old. [78]

Although oral contraceptives (birth control pills) are frequently recommended and prescribed, they may actually increase insulin resistance, making a woman less tolerant of carbohydrates and increasing triglycerides, leading to higher levels of cardiovascular disease. Additionally, there is a two-fold increase in cardiovascular events in woman with PCOS who take oral contraceptives versus normal women. [78]

PCOS Treatment

Weight loss significantly improves symptoms of PCOS. Even a five percent loss of body weight is enough to improve clinical symptoms of PCOS.[65] A carbohydrate controlled diet with protein, monounsaturated and omega-3 rich fats at each meal and snack can significantly calm down insulin resistance leading to weight loss.

It is important to include omega-3 rich foods and/or supplements as needed. The three types of omega-3 fatty acids – Alpha Linolenic Acid (ALA), Eicosapentaenoic Acid (EPA), and Docosahexaenoic Acid (DHA) – become extremely important in women with PCOS for hormone balance (see *Fat chapter* for more info on omega-3). Both EPA and DHA are found in fish and fish oil. One tablespoon per day of ground flax seed is recommended to achieve two grams of ALA per day, and between 500-1000 mg. each of DHA and EPA is recommended to help with symptoms of PCOS. If an individual consumes fish several times a week, a supplement may not be necessary.

A drug given with PCOS is *Metformin* also called *Glucophage*. Metformin is an insulin-sensitizing drug that lowers insulin resistance and can assist with lowering appetite and weight and normalizing hormone levels. Side effects of Metformin can include gas, bloating and diarrhea, which can be exacerbated by a high-carbohydrate diet. If a woman modifies her carbohydrate intake, these symptoms may be minimized or nonexistent.

Although PCOS can be a challenging condition to diagnose and treat, there are many lifestyle and medication treatments available. Even modest weight loss can significantly alter symptoms of PCOS. Changing your diet, in addition to exercise and activity are extremely helpful with lowering insulin resistance and assisting with weight loss.

A carbohydrate controlled diet along with omega-3 rich fats has been shown to be extremely successful in treating PCOS. Metformin is the drug of choice in helping to lower insulin resistance, cardiovascular symptoms and assisting with hormone balance.

PCOS does not need to define an individual nor control their lives. With proper self care, you can conquer the challenges and live a healthy balanced life.

Cancer

Cancer is the second largest cause of death in the U.S., coming in behind heart disease.[80] Research over the last few years has consistently linked high insulin levels to development of certain types of cancers and cancer reoccurrence. **A high glycemic carbohydrate diet can increase production of insulin, which in turn can increase cell growth of tumors in the body.** When insulin levels are high, tumor cells can get the food they need to divide and multiply.

Is there a connection between carbohydrates and cancer?

Pancreatic cancer
A group of researchers examined the records of 89,000 women participating in the Nurses' Health study in 2002. They found that women of normal weight who ate large amounts of refined starches, such as white bread and potatoes, slightly increased their risk of pancreatic cancer. Women who were overweight, did not get a lot of exercise, and ate a lot of starchy foods were 2.5 times more likely to develop pancreatic cancer than if they ate other types of healthy carbohydrates. [81]

One of the co-authors of the study, Charles S. Fuchs, discussed how replacing starchy foods that increase insulin levels with healthy carbohydrates

from fruits and vegetables can improve your health by not only lowering risk of cancer, but diabetes and cardiovascular disease as well.

Other expert opinions
Richard Bergman, Ph.D., chair of the Department of Physiology and Biophysics at USC, is considered an expert in the field of insulin and has linked high insulin levels to diabetes, high blood pressure, cardiovascular disease and cancer. [82]

C-peptide, insulin and cancer connection
At the December 2007 American Association for Cancer Research Sixth Annual Conference, research was presented showing women with diabetes are one and a half times more likely to develop colorectal cancer than women who do not have diabetes.

Further studies presented showed that among women with invasive breast cancer who had elevated c-peptide levels (a measure for amount of insulin secretion), the risk of death was three times as high as the risk of death with women with normal c-peptides. The researchers stated that these results could show that both insulin and c-peptides levels are possible markers for breast cancer diagnosis.

Esophageal cancer
A 2008 study at Case Western Reserve University found a strong correlation between increased total carbohydrate intake and rising esophageal cancer rates.[83] The link was mostly in those consuming refined carbohydrates in the form of corn syrup. The authors of this research state their study shows evidence for the link between carbohydrate intake, obesity and insulin resistance.

Alcohol and cancer
Published in the *International Journal of Cancer*, a 2007 study done in the UK looked at the alcohol intake of 480,000 people over a six-year period.[84]

The study showed that those who drank more than 30 grams per day of alcohol (about 2.5 drinks) had approximately a 25 percent increase in colon and rectal cancers. One drink is approximately equal to 5 ounces of wine, 1.5 ounces of hard liquor, or 12 ounces of beer, which can also be thought of as a serving of carbohydrate.

Multiple studies exist on the link between alcohol intake and breast cancer risk. Wendy Chen, M.D., Ph.D., a cancer specialist at the Dana-Farber Cancer Institute in Boston, presented her research data at the annual meeting of the American Society of Clinical Oncology in 2005. Her study tracked the health of 122,000 women since 1976 who were free of cancer when the study began. [85]

When compared with those who did not drink, they discovered the following:

- Women who drank the equivalent of half a glass of wine a day were 6 percent more likely to develop breast cancer

- Women who drank the equivalent of a glass or two of wine per day had a 21 percent increased risk of breast cancer

- Women who drank the equivalent of two drinks per day had a 37 percent increased risk of cancer

Alcohol can increase breast cancer risk since it:

- Increases blood triglyceride levels

- Increases estrogen levels in blood circulation

- Decreases the liver's processing of excess estrogen in the blood and decreases immune function. [86]

A 2009 study published in the UK in the Journal of the National Cancer Institute showed similar results in women consuming alcohol: consuming as little as one drink per day increases a woman's risk of several types of cancer by 13 percent. [87]

Everyone reads about how a glass of red wine per day is good for your health. However, the studies that have looked at the correlation between wine and health have consistently shown that resveratrol is the component of alcohol which prevents disease, which is not in the fruit of the grape, but is contained in the skins. Therefore, just eating some grapes every day with skins can be more beneficial to health than a glass of wine.

Weight and cancer

In 2007, a major report called *Food, Nutrition, Physical Activity, and the Prevention of Cancer: A Global Perspective* was published linking cancer to diet, physical activity, and weight. The most profound finding of the report linked excess body fat to six types of cancer, including colon, kidney, pancreas, and adenocarcinoma of the esophagus and endometrium and post-menopausal breast cancer.

Walter Willett, M.D., a co-author of the study stated that, "Obesity is approaching smoking as a cancer risk."

Some of the recommendations of the report include maintaining your weight within a normal range, being physically active everyday, eating foods of plant origin, and limiting alcohol and salt.

Summary: Cancer and Diet

Clearly some types of cancer have strong correlations with high insulin levels, which can be caused by high levels of carbohydrates in the diet, including refined and starchy grains and alcohol intake. Of course there are many other causes and cures of cancer, which are beyond the scope of this book. However, the message is still clear: eating healthy forms of carbohydrate such as vegetables and fruits not only keep insulin levels normal, but provide the important antioxidants and phytochemicals our body needs to maintain a healthy immune system. Getting healthy sources of omega-3 fatty acids to lower inflammation in the body, lowering your intake of omega-6 fatty acids (see *Fat chapter*), and getting regular exercise are all essential to good health.

Hypertension and Heart Disease

Research clearly shows that high blood pressure can be brought on by weight. The Joint National Committee on prevention, evaluation and treatment of high blood pressure published a report in 2003 that stated:

"Weight reduction in overweight or obese individuals can reduce systolic blood pressure by 5-20 mmHg for every 10 kg. (about 22 pounds) of body weight lost."[88]

The **DASH** (Dietary Approaches to Stop Hypertension) diet has been well studied over the last several years with respect to its effect on blood pressure. The DASH diet is rich in vegetables, fruits, low-fat dairy, and nuts. It limits total fat, sodium, and alcohol. The DASH diet has been shown to reduce blood pressure by 8-14 mmHg. For example, if your blood pressure is 140/95, losing weight or altering your diet could lower your blood pressure to a range of 120-135/75-90 respectively without medication.

A 2008 study published in the *Archives of Internal Medicine* used the Nurses' Health Study database to transform existing diet intake questionnaires into a DASH-style diet score. The goal of the study was to examine the relationship between diet and incidental causes of heart attacks, strokes, or cardiac-related death during 24 years of follow-up.

The study looked at eight diet components of 88,000 women – fruits, vegetables, nuts and legumes, whole grains, low-fat dairy, sodium, red and processed meats, and sweetened beverages. A higher DASH style score resulted in a lower incidence of cardiac and stroke-related events – an almost inverse relationship. [89]

Here again, we see how the diet can lower *inflammation* in the body, which in turn can lower blood pressure, heart disease and cardiac-related effects. It is astounding how simply changing your diet, even without weight loss, can help in disease prevention.

Weight, exercise and diet modifications undoubtedly lower health issues, including high blood pressure and heart disease.

What about heart disease? Clearly lowering *inflammation* through diet and exercise has a profound effect on lowering heart disease in most forms. In 2008, researchers at the University of Michigan looked at cardiometabolic abnormalities, including blood pressure, triglycerides, fasting blood sugars and c-reactive protein in 5,400 subjects. [90]

The most striking finding was that those with the lowest fitness level were four times more likely to die than those with the highest level of fitness. Activity had a huge effect on whether the individuals had markers of heart disease or not.

Diet has been well researched and studies clearly indicate that a diet in the form of high glycemic carbohydrates is linked to fatty liver, since carbohydrate that is not metabolized or stored as fat gets shuttled to the liver. When the liver cannot store additional carbohydrates, it produces triglycerides.

High triglycerides are linked to heart disease and stroke. The same type of diet proves itself in this arena as well – carbohydrates in the form of fruits and veggies, nuts, seeds, healthy sources of proteins, and fats, including omega-3 rich foods.

In addition, a 5-10 percent loss of body weight has been reported to improve the cholesterol panel, insulin sensitivity, endothelial function, as well as reduce thrombosis and inflammatory makers. [91]

Clearly, changing your diet and exercise regime will lower *inflammation*, which can lower your blood pressure and risk of heart disease.

So what about your cholesterol panel?

If you go to your internist or family practice doctor once a year, they will usually perform a physical. This will involve routine blood work, which includes a cholesterol panel. The different components of the cholesterol panel and how they relate to food intake are as follows:

- total cholesterol

- LDL cholesterol

- HDL cholesterol

- triglycerides

- ratio (total cholesterol/HDL)

It is routinely recommended that **total cholesterol** be less than 200. However, the most essential part of the cholesterol panel may be the other parts that point to issues with heart disease. Sometimes, a person can have a perfect cholesterol panel with ideal numbers and still have plaque in the arteries. Conversely, someone can have high levels of cholesterol with clean arteries. A conscientious physician will order other tests run on his or her patients to rule out any problems.

LDL cholesterol stands for *low-density lipoprotein cholesterol*, which is classically known as the "lousy" or bad cholesterol. There are several types of LDL cholesterol – a discussion of which is beyond the scope of this book. Suffice it to say that for a lower risk of heart disease, an LDL of less than 100 is recommended. Recently, guidelines came out that a person should have an LDL less than 70, which is a difficult to achieve unless you are taking cholesterol medication. Increased amounts of trans fat in the diet are associated with increasing LDL cholesterol and heart disease.

HDL cholesterol stands for *high-density lipoprotein cholesterol,* also known as the "happy" or good cholesterol. HDL is sort of a scrubbing agent that rids the body of bad cholesterol. So, the higher number of HDL the better (greater than 50 is recommended). Low HDL cholesterol (approximately less than 40) is associated with insulin resistance or metabolic syndrome and an increased risk of heart disease.

Triglycerides are the storage form of fat and are associated with carbohydrate sensitivity in the body. The liver is the organ that decides what to do when glucose is transported there. Either it is stored as glycogen (chains of glucose) in the muscles, used for energy or turned into triglycerides. For example, if one has metabolic syndrome and/or carbohydrate sensitivity, there is often an increased level of triglycerides. An ideal level is below 150. If your triglycerides are in the 200-1,000 range, it is associated with carbohydrate sensitivity. The wonderful thing about triglycerides is that they are very responsive to dietary changes. By decreasing carbohydrate intake, typically from starches and alcohol, we can see a drop to almost normal levels in six to eight weeks. Changes in cholesterol are much more sluggish and take time to respond to dietary changes.

The **ratio** is the level of total cholesterol divided by

the HDL. It is ideal to have a ratio of less than four since ratios greater than four are associated with an increased risk of heart disease. Having a high HDL is advantageous since it lowers the ratio.

Ratio = Total Cholesterol/HDL

Poor ratio: 160/30 = 5.3

Good Ratio: 220/75 = 2.9

For example, one can have what seems like a low total cholesterol level such as 160, but if that is paired with an HDL of 30, the ratio is 5.3. Conversely, one can have a total cholesterol of 220 with an HDL of 75, making the ratio 2.9. Look at and assess all the values and how they go together. Taking one number out of context does not give the whole picture with respect to someone's health.

The Berkeley Heart Lab in California is considered the best in the world for tests with breakdowns in the types of LDL and other pertinent blood work related to risks of heart disease. If you have a family history of heart disease, it might be worth sending your blood to this lab to be analyzed.

Several researchers in the field of cardiology have shown that testing cholesterol values may soon be a thing of the past. Recent research has shown that a value known as **Apo B** is a better indicator of the appearance of the atherosclerotic process (i.e. plaque in the arteries) than the cholesterol value, and a more accurate measure of the risk of vascular disease than measuring LDL cholesterol.

Apo B is the primary substance that is responsible for carrying cholesterol to the tissues, which can lead to plaque and eventually heart disease. Studies show weight loss can significantly lower Apo B production by the liver.

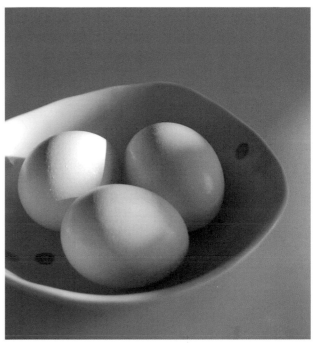

Eggs: high in protein and lutein

Cholesterol: egg the question, or egg to differ?

Myth: Eating eggs in your diet will increase your blood cholesterol levels.

Fact: Stephen B. Kritchevsky, M.D., from the Wake Forest University School of Medicine and J. Paul Sticht Center on Aging states in his 2004 review on eggs:

> *"Data from free-living populations show that egg consumption is not associated with higher cholesterol levels. Furthermore, as a whole, the epidemiological literature does not support the data that egg consumption is a risk for coronary disease."* [92]

Very few studies exist linking any connection between cholesterol levels in the diet and cholesterol levels in the blood. When the guidelines were made up by the various health boards recommending a limit to cholesterol levels, it was based more on common sense than on research. It does make sense that if a food contains cholesterol, it must increase the blood cholesterol value. However, this analogy never really panned out.

Egg Study 1

In 1999, a study came out that linked egg consumption to risk of cardiovascular disease only in diabetic men. Otherwise, the group concluded that having an egg a day is unlikely to have any impact on risk of cardiovascular disease or stroke in healthy subjects. [93]

Egg Study 2

In 2007, a group of researchers at Zeenat Qureshi Stroke Research center in Newark, New Jersey, studied 10,000 adults and categorized them into three categories:

1. Those consuming **less than one egg** per week

2. Those consuming **one to six eggs** per week

3. Those consuming **greater than six eggs** per week

After adjusting for age differences, there was no significant difference found between those who ate less than one egg per week compared to those who ate six eggs or more per week. The researchers concluded that eating more than six eggs per week does not increase risk of coronary heart disease or stroke. [94]

Egg Study 3

In 2008, a study came out that looked at the relationship between egg consumption and risk of heart disease as part of the Physicians' Health Study (a long-term study using physicians as patients to research multiple health issues). [95] They found that egg consumption of up to six times per week was not associated with heart failure, but greater than seven eggs per week was associated with an increased rate of heart failure, which seemed stronger among diabetics. However, the study did not take into account the subjects overall lifestyle, including the composition of the diet.

To egg or not to egg?

Eggs are an excellent source of protein, and most of the fat contained in the egg is polyunsaturated and monounsaturated fat. It is an excellent source of the antioxidant lutein, which can lower certain inflammatory responses in the body.

Bruce Griffin, Ph.D., a researcher from the University of Surrey, stated in *Nutrition Bulletin* in February 2009:

> *"The link between egg consumption and raised cholesterol levels, which ultimately could lead to cardiovascular disease, was based on out-of-date information. The egg is a nutrient-dense food, a valuable source of high-quality protein and essential nutrients that is not high in saturated fat or energy… it is high time we dispelled the mythology surrounding eggs and heart disease and restored them to their rightful place on our menus where they can make a valuable contribution to healthy balanced diets."* [96]

Eating an egg daily or two eggs several times a week easily fits in with a healthy lifestyle and is even beneficial. If you are diabetic, it might be prudent to limit your intake to less than seven eggs per week, taking into consideration all the studies on eggs. So, don't be afraid of eggs, or limit yourself to egg whites. Enjoy an omelet and get on with life!

Arthritis

While there are no proven diets for arthritis, lowering *inflammation* can be helpful in relieving symptoms associated with arthritis. Maintaining a healthy weight is essential since every additional pound can increase pressure on the joints by 8-10 pounds.

Balance in the diet is critical, and minimizing starchy and refined carbohydrates is essential, since they are associated with increasing *inflammation.* Increasing intake of omega-3 rich fats and lowering intake of omega-6 fats (*see Fat chapter*) is helpful in lowering inflammation in the body.

In 2000, Joel Kremer, M.D., professor of medicine and head of Rheumatology at Albany Medical College in New York, reviewed 17 randomized, controlled clinical trials assessing the pain relieving effects of omega-3 fatty acid supplementation in patients with rheumatoid arthritis.[97] The paper summarized that taking approximately 3,000 mg. per day of both DHA and EPA for over 12 weeks, in addition to their regular medication, had a significant decrease in morning stiffness and joint tenderness in rheumatoid arthritis patients.

In my practice, I have seen patients with all forms of arthritis benefit greatly from weight loss, rebalancing their diets with minimal processed foods and increased amounts of omega-3 rich fats. In addition, regular exercise and activity has been shown to help alleviate symptoms of arthritis.

Osteoporosis

Osteoporosis is a condition in which the density of your bones decreases since more bone cells are lost than replaced with aging. According to the International Osteoporosis Foundation, it affects 1 in 3 women and 1 in 5 men.

The two nutritional components most important in maintaining good bone health are calcium and vitamin D. Bone tissue is made of calcium, and vitamin D is important for the development and maintenance of bone. (See *Vitamin chapter* for more information on calcium and vitamin D needs.) Studies indicate that vitamin D not only assists with absorption of calcium, but seems to be related to less likelihood for falling down or fractures in bones if you fall.

A 2007 study done at Harvard looked at 57,000 subjects and intake of vitamin D supplements over a 5.7 year period. Results showed that for those with heart disease, taking additional vitamin D was linked to lower levels of mortality. Risk reduction was 7-8 percent and was greater in those who took supplements for at least three years. [98] Therefore, obtaining adequate vitamin D from either sunshine, food or a vitamin pill is not only linked to bone health, but can play an important role in longevity.

Obtaining adequate calcium intake from your diet is vitally important as well. Several recipes in the recipe section of the book incorporate dairy as an easy way to achieve your calcium needs.

GERD

Gastroesophageal reflux disease (GERD) is a chronic condition affecting 44 percent of the American population at least once a month, with daily occurrences affecting about 7 percent of the population.[99] Acid reflux happens when stomach acid and juices travel back from the stomach into the esophagus. The muscle between the two organs called the esophageal sphincter may be relaxed or not close tightly, which causes the reflux. Certain foods have been related to GERD since it is thought that they relax this muscle. These foods are:

- coffee
- alcohol
- chocolate
- peppermint
- pepper
- spicy foods
- onions and garlic

Other strategies for minimizing symptoms associated with GERD are:

- Eating small, frequent meals every 2-3 hours
- Avoiding tight garments to decrease compression on the abdomen

Many modalities exist for trying to assist with reflux and heartburn, some which may work on addressing the symptom but do not really address the cause of GERD.

Consuming a lot of refined starches and large amounts of grains without having the capacity to utilize these foods causes symptoms to develop. For those with insulin resistance, if their bodies do not metabolize the carbohydrates they are consuming in a timely fashion, either because they are insulin resistant or their body cannot keep up with the amount of carbohydrate they are taking in, GERD can be a natural consequence. The carbohydrate can produce gas, which will put pressure on the sphincter muscle/value and cause reflux.

In my practice, I have seen multiple cases of reflux completely resolve within a week or two by rebalancing the diet with more protein, a moderate amount of carbohydrate and good sources of fat. If rebalancing the diet or weight loss does not eliminate symptoms of reflux, then using regular modalities of lowering foods linked to reflux, spicy foods, and increasing exercise may be required.

Summary: Prevention is Power

The research clearly shows a correlation between diet and chronic, low-grade *inflammation*. If you don't want a low-grade fever going on in your body, changing your diet is essential. Besides balancing your diet with healthy carbohydrates, protein at each meal and healthy fats, include an abundance of anti-inflammatory foods with phytonutrients (outlined in the *Phytochemical chapter*). Including colorful foods high in carotenoids, polyphenols and other phytonutrients can keep many forms of disease away. You really do have a choice in how your health plays out.

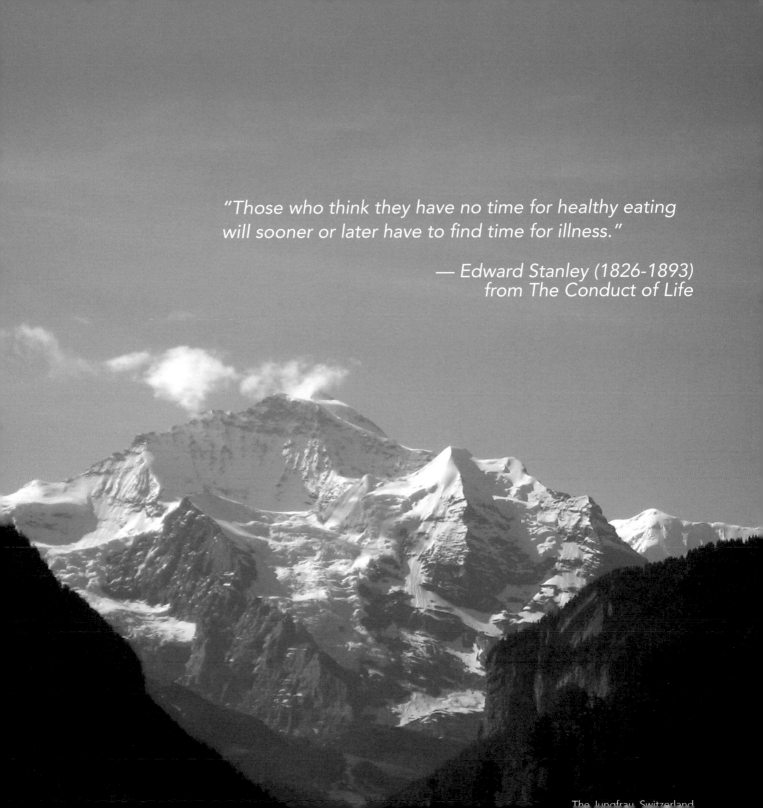

"*Those who think they have no time for healthy eating will sooner or later have to find time for illness.*"

— *Edward Stanley (1826-1893)*
from The Conduct of Life

The Jungfrau, Switzerland

Medications and Your Weight

Often clients come in for a consult due to their concern about weight gain. Their stories are similar. They have been at a certain weight for many years and suddenly they gain weight for no apparent reason. They were not eating more or changing their exercise patterns. After an analysis of their food history, I inquire if they are taking medications. It is not unusual to see weight gain coincide with the onset of a drug. A light bulb goes off in their heads, and they realize the weight gain was not all their fault.

Weight is multi-factorial. Weight loss or gain is caused by complex groups of systems in our bodies, with influential factors such as genetics, hormones, stress, lack of sleep, and yes, medications. Medications may be necessary for a variety of reasons, but can cause other issues such as weight gain.

Linda, a young mother, came to my office after being referred by her physician. All her life she had been tall and thin, even after having two children. Six months prior to our consultation, she encountered difficulties in her life and became depressed. Her physician put her on Paxil, which is an antidepressant known as a selective serotonin reuptake inhibitor (SSRI). Within a few months, she had gained 60 pounds, and although she was less depressed, she became very uncomfortable in her body, and the depression returned.

Although her diet was not stellar, it was not cause for a 60-pound weight gain. Initially, Linda stayed on the drug and worked on her food and exercise regimen. When it became apparent her weight was not budging, she decided the depression had lightened and she was ready to cease taking the medication. Together with her physician, she was weaned off the drug. She fine-tuned her diet and exercise program. It took about nine months, but she resumed her normal, slender body.

Linda, like many others, has discovered there are different classifications of drugs which can cause weight gain for a variety of reasons.

Antidepressants

Selective serotonin reuptake inhibitors are one class of antidepressants also known as SSRIs. These are commonly known as Prozac, Zoloft, Paxil, Luvox, Celexa, and Lexapro. SSRIs can cause a loss of appetite with some weight loss initially. However, after the first six months of taking SSRIs, weight gain is common. Weight gains of 10-40 pounds are not uncommon, due to increased carbohydrate cravings that are the result of insulin resistance caused by taking the drugs over an extended period of time.

Most clients in my practice do not lose weight for several months even after they cease their medications. This is because insulin resistance requires time to calm and reverse before the person's natural metabolism resumes.

Serotonin-Norepinephrine Reuptake Inhibitors (SNRIs) are another class of antidepressants and are commonly known as Cymbalta, Effexor, and Pristiq. These drugs can still cause weight gain, but not to the same degree SSRIs have in increasing insulin resistance and weight gain.

Tricyclic antidepressants, also known as TCAs, are an older classification of drugs that were more commonly prescribed before SSRIs came into practice. TCAs include Elavil, Pamelor or Aventyl, Sinequan or Adapin, Ascendin, Tofranil or Janimine, Norpramine or Pertofrane, Anafranil, Rhotramine or Surmontil, Vivactil, and Ludiomil. Weight gain is a common and a well-known adverse affect of short-term and long-term treatment with tricyclic antidepressants, primarily as a result of excessive appetite. [100,101] Because TCAs have more side effects; they are not prescribed as commonly as SSRIs.

Monamine oxidase inhibitors, also known as MAOIs, are also an older classification of antidepressants and commonly named Nardil, Parnate, Manerix, Humoryl, Marplan. MAOIs can cause weight gain in the short- and long term. Unfortunately, if you are taking MAOIs, you will need to restrict foods high in tyramine. This group of drugs can cause tyramine to increase. If someone is taking these drugs and gets a sudden flood of tyramine in the blood stream, it can cause a fatal increase in blood pressure, which can burst blood vessels in the brain.

Tyramine is commonly found in foods that are aged, fermented or spoiled. Foods that should be avoided are all aged and mature cheeses, sausages, salami, smoked or pickled fish, overripe or fermented fruits, any soups containing meat extracts or foods with meat tenderizers, tap beer and limited alcohol. Since these medications limit choices in the diet, they are not commonly prescribed.

Several other antidepressants that do not fall under the other classifications are Remeron, Serzone, Trazadone, and Wellbutrin. Remeron has been associated with significant weight gain. [102] Serzone or Trazadone are unlikely to have much effect on weight. Wellbutrin is weight neutral and has even been shown to increase weight loss.

Anticonvulsants

Anticonvulsants that are currently available are Depakote, Tegretol, Neurontin, Lamictal, and Topamex. Anticonvulsants can increase appetite and insulin resistance leading to weight gain. Depakote is linked to the largest weight gains, with Neurontin and Tegretol falling slightly behind. Lamictal seems weight neutral and Topamex has been linked to lowering the appetite and weight loss.

Conventional Mood Stabilizers

Mood stabilizers are regularly used with treatment of bipoloar disorder. Lithium is associated with weight gain. Although weight gain with Lithium is less common than Depakote, one third to two thirds of patients treated with Lithium gain weight, and 25 percent gain enough weight to be classified as obese. [102]

Anti-psychotic Medications

Anti-psychotic medications include Haldol, Abilify, Prolixin, Mellaril, Clozaril, Zyprexa, Seroquel,

Risperdal, and Serlect. Some have been linked to increased appetite. Clozaril and Zyprexa have been associated with the greatest weight gain, followed by Risperdal, and less with the other drugs.

Corticosteroids

If you are taking prednisone for an inflammatory condition or an allergic reaction, it can affect your weight. Corticosteroids can result in weight gain through an increased appetite and carbohydrate cravings. Sometimes it may feel like the appetite is insatiable.

Large doses of corticosteroids can also increase fluid retention, creating a bloated puffy feeling though the body, which is evident in the face, commonly called a moon face. The moon face generally happens with those who need to take corticosteroids for long periods of time or indefinitely, such as with organ transplant recipients. Insulin resistance is almost always an issue with these drugs.

Beta-blockers and Diuretics

Older generation beta blockers prescribed to treat high blood pressure can be associated with weight gain. Inderal, Lopressor or Toprol XL and Tenormin, in addition to some diuretics, are associated with weight gain of at least 2-5 pounds. These drugs are among the agents recommended for first-line therapy for hypertension, yet these medications increase the risk of insulin resistance or metabolic syndrome. [103]

The mechanism is not clearly understood, but it is thought these drugs lower the metabolic rate by about 1-2 percent, which can affect weight over time. Some research shows beta-blockers can exacerbate insulin resistance.

Diabetic Medications

There are many different types of diabetic drugs, and several types can increase weight. Sulfonylureas are the oldest class of diabetic medication and include drugs such as Glucotrol, Diabeta, Micronase, or Glynase, Amaryl, Diabinese, and Orinase. These drugs increase insulin production from the pancreas which can increase appetite and weight.

Thiozolidinediones (called TZD's) such as Avandia or Actos are a class of drugs that can cause fluid retention and weight gain through an increase in appetite. With diabetes, when blood sugars are elevated, the food may not be properly utilized. In taking a drug such as Actos or Avandia, a person is better able to utilize the food that is broken down to sugar or glucose. If an individual is taking in more food than he needs, weight gain will result.

Birth Control Pills

Hormones are a complex topic that is beyond the scope of this book. Oral contraceptives can increase insulin resistance in some women, which can increase carbohydrate cravings and appetite leading to weight gain. The incidence of weight gain can depend on the women's genetics and the type of pill that is prescribed.

Summary: Medications

If you are currently taking any drugs that are associated with weight gain, do not take yourself off these drugs without the supervision and assistance of your physician. Because a drug is associated with weight gain does not mean you will automatically experience this effect in your body since reactions vary.

Being attentive to your diet and exercise program can negate the effect of a drug on your weight. Other times, the drug is necessary for your health and happiness despite the weight gain. Discuss your concerns with your physician, and if you are gaining weight due to one of these drugs, consider a visit to a registered dietitian to optimize your nutrition and exercise regimen as an initial plan for your health.

Keeping you safe

For any type of medication, it is important to closely follow the orders of your physician and discuss how to take the drug, the duration, and how to wean off the drug when necessary. Many physicians work closely with registered dietitians to help with the side effects of medications. If you have questions about a drug you may be taking, or if it is affecting your weight, please communicate your concerns to your physician before making any changes.

Closing Thoughts: A Lifelong Journey

Do you know those children's books where you have to find the hidden character throughout the book? Within these pages is the not-so-hidden message to eat a healthy balance of nutrients and to exercise. Perhaps self-prevention is the best and most powerful tool we have to fight against disease.

At the beginning of the book, I talked about goals and the key success factors of *motivation* and *importance* in making lifestyle modifications that last. The clients I've worked with who are the most successful in achieving their health goals have embraced both of these ingredients for change.

Martin was a patient who was referred by his doctor for weight management and high cholesterol. He was highly motivated and recognized the importance of changing his lifestyle. I want to leave you with his story, as I think it illustrates the rewards that can come with taking charge of your health. I hope you find his words as inspiring as I do.

Martin's Journey

I had wanted to change my life for a long time. It was something I had an external and internal impetus to do. It's something I've needed and resisted, probably to avoid facing the traumatic events of my childhood, which included pain and fear. Because of this, I accepted a number of debilitating conditions as part of my everyday life, including obesity, anxiety, depression, poor relationship skills, and fatigue. I was living below my true potential, ultimately out of lack of love for myself.

After being diagnosed with adult ADD/ ADHD, I began treatment, and the pieces of the puzzle began falling into place. I started dealing with the medical issues that had been daunting me. I started working out on a regular basis, with the combination of a high-powered gym and a daily workout routine.

As a next step, I knew I wanted to see a nutritionist, and my physician recommended Susan. This referral turned out to be most fortuitous.

Working with Susan, we were able to isolate my food addiction and establish a diet that literally had pounds melting off my body. In five months, I lost 50 pounds and achieved a stable weight of 195 pounds. After achieving this weight loss, I reached higher levels of mindfulness and relaxation. With my increased activity and better nutrition, my energy levels increased. I felt healthier, attractive and more accomplished than ever before.

The dramatic changes I went through were the beginning of a lifelong journey. Healthy eating and exercise helped with the transition to dealing with my core issues. This change gave me the unique opportunity to realize my goals, begin to reach my potential, and in turn, bring positive change to the big, wide world.

We all have our own motivations and reasons for lifestyle change. Our ingredients may vary, but they all add up to a recipe for life. I wish you every success on your journey to good health.

Susan

References and Index

References

1. Ludwig, DS., M.D. (February 10, 2006) "Glycemic Foods and Obesity"; Presented at the 53rd Postgraduate ADA Advanced Postgraduate Course. San Francisco, CA.

2. Willett, WC. and Stampfer, Meir J. (December 17, 2002) "Rebuilding the Pyramid"; *Scientific American*.

3. Lutsey, PL., et. al. (February 12, 2008) "Dietary intake and the development of metabolic syndrome. The atherosclerosis risk in communities study"; *Circulation*. 117(6):754-61.

4. Swithers, SE., and Davidson, TL. (2008) "A role for sweet taste: calorie predictive relations in energy regulation in rats"; *Behavioral Neuroscience*. Vol. 122(1):161-173.

5. International Food Information Council: "Metabolic syndrome: lifestyle strikes again"; *Food Insight May/June 2002*.

6. Neel JV. (1962) "Diabetes mellitus: a thrifty genotype rendered detrimental by progress?"; *The American Journal of Human Genetics*. 14:353–62.

7. Leidy HJ, et al. (2009) "Increased dietary protein consumed at breakfast leads to an initial and sustained feeling of fullness during energy restriction compared to other meal times"; *British Journal of Nutrition*. 101(6):798-803.

8. Mattes, R. Human Hunger. (Summer 1999) *SCAN's Pulse*. p. 16-17.

9. Batterham, RL. et al. (2006) "Critical role of peptide YY in protein-mediated satiation and body-weight regulation"; *Cell Metabolism*. 4(3):223-233.

10. Foster-Schubert, KE., Cummings, DE. et al. (2008) "Acyl and Total Ghrelin are strongly suppressed by ingested protein, weakly by lipids and biphasically by carbohydrates"; *Journal of Endocrinology and Metabolism*. 93(5):1971-9.

11. Westerterp- Plantenga, MS. (November 2003) "The significance of protein in food intake and body weight regulation"; *Clinical Nutrition and Metabolic Care*. 6(6):635-638.

12. Johnston, CS., et. al. (2002) "Postprandial thermogeneis is increased by 100% on a high-protein, low-fat diet versus a high-carbohydrate, low-fat diet in healthy, young women"; *Journal of the American College of Nutrition*. Feb:21(1):55-61.

13. Campbell, WW., Trappe, TA., Wolfe, RR., Evans, WJ. (2001) "The recommended dietary allowance for protein may not be adequate for older people to maintain skeletal muscle"; *Journal of Gerontology Biological Sciences and Medical Sciences*. 56:M373 –M380.

14. Campbell WW, Evans WJ. et. al. (1995) "Effects of resistance training and dietary protein intake on protein metabolism in older adults"; *American Journal of Physiological Endocrinology and Metabolism*. 268 (6):E1143-E1153.

15. Mannenen, A. (2004) "High protein weight loss diets and purported adverse effects: where is the evidence?"; *Sports Nutrition Review Journal* 1(1):45-51.

16. Dawson-Hughes, B. (March 2003). "Interaction of dietary calcium and protein in bone health in humans"; *Journal of Nutrition*. 122:852S-854S.

17. Gannon, MC. (2003) "An increase in dietary protein improves the blood glucose response in person with type 2 diabetes"; *American Journal of Clinical Nutrition*. 78(4): 734-741.

18. Lemley, B. (February 2004) "What does science say you should eat?"; *Discover*. p. 43-49.

19. Castelli, W. (July 1992) *Archives of Internal Medicine*, 152:7:1371-1372.

20. Multiple Risk Factor Intervention Trial Research Group. "Multiple risk factor intervention trial. Risk factor changes and mortality results"; *Journal of the American Medical Association*.1982, 248:1465-77.

21. Tavazzi, L. et. al. (2008) "Statins and the Omega-3 fatty acid supplementation in heart failure." *Lancet*, 372(9645):1223-30.

22. Willett, WC. www.bantransfat.com – statement from Dr. Willett regarding banning trans fat from restaurant food.

23. Vinikoor, LC.,et. al. (2008) "Consumption of trans-fatty acid and its association with colorectal adenomas"; *American Journal of Epidemiology*. 168(3):289-297.

24. Kleiner, SM. (1999) "Water: an essential but overlooked nutrient"; *Journal of the American Dietetic Association*. 99:200-206.

25. Chan, J., et.al. (2002) "Water, other Fluids, and fatal coronary heart disease: the adventist health study"; *American Journal of Epidemiology*. 155 (9):827-833.

26. Nestle, M. *What to Eat* (2006) New York: North Point Press.

27. Mercola.com. (2007) "The dangers of MSG".

28. Sheehan, D., and Doerge, D. (February 18, 1999) "Scientists protest soy approval"; *Letter to the FDA*.

29. Fallon, S., and Enig, M. (2000) *Tragedy & Hype: The Third International Soy Symposium*. p. 1-17.

30. Drewett, RF. (2007) "The social facilitation of food intake"; *Archives of Disease in Childhood*. 92:377.

31. Racette SB., et al. (2008) "Influence of weekend lifestyle patterns on body weight"; *Obesity*. August 16(8):1826-30.

32. Beck, JS. (2007) *The Beck Diet Solution*. Birmingham: Oxmoor House.

33. Wansink, B. (2007) *Mindless Eating: Why We Eat More Than We Think*. New York: Bantam Books.

34. Berg, F. (1995) "The Biology of Human Starvation"; *Health Risks of Weight Loss*. p. 140-145.

35. Kratina, K., and King, NL. (July/August 1996) "Hunger and satiety: helping clients get in touch with their body signals"; *Healthy Weight Journal*. p. 68-71.

36. Mellin, L. (1997) *The Solution*. New York: Regan Books.

37. Sease, JM. (January 2009) "Does vitamin B12 help relieve fatigue?"; *Medscape*.

38. Cannell, J., and Hollis, B. (November 1, 2008) "The use of vitamin D in clinical practice"; *Alternative Medicine Review*. 13(1):6-20.

39. Autier, P., et al. (2007) "Vitamin D supplementation and total mortality: a meta-analysis of randomized controlled trials"; *Archives of Internal Medicine*, 167:1730-1737.

40. Gombart, A. (2005) "CAMP gene is a direct target of the vitamin D receptor and is

strongly up-regulated in myeloid cells by 1,25 dihydroxyvitamin D3"; *FASEB* J. Jul:19 (9): 1067-77.

41. Clark, LC., et. al. (1996) "Effects of selenium supplementation for cancer prevention in patients with carcinoma of the skin. A randomized controlled trial"; Nutritional Prevention of Cancer Study Group. *Journal of the American Medical Association*. Dec 25:276(24):1957-63.

42. Mossad, SB., et. al. (July 1996) "Zinc gluconate lozenges for treating the common cold"; *Annals of Internal Medicine*. 125(2):81-88.

43. Liu, RH., et. al. (2007) "Triterpenoids isolated from apple peels have potent antiproliferative activity and may be partially responsible for apple's anticancer activity"; *Journal of Agricultural and Food Chemistry*. 55(11):4366-4370.

44. Di Giuseppe, R., et. al. (2008) "Regular consumption of dark chocolate is associated with low serum concentrations of c-reactive protein in a healthy Italian population"; *Journal of Nutrition*. 138, Issue 10:1939-1945.

45. Nieman, DC., et. al. (2000) "Immune function in female elite rowers and nonathletes"; *British Journal of Sports Medicine*. 34:181-187.

46. Nieman, DC., et. al. (2006) "Relationship between salivary IgA secretion and upper respiratory tract infection following a 160-km race"; *Journal of Sports Medicine and Physical Fitness*. 46:158-162.

47. Shors, TJ. (March 2009) "Saving New Brain Cells"; *Scientific American*, p. 47-54.

48. Knowler, WC., et. al. (2002) "Reduction in the incidence of type 2 diabetes with lifestyle intervention or metformin"; *New England Journal of Medicine*. 346(6):393-403.

49. Lee, IM., et. al. (2001) "Physical activity and coronary heart disease in women: is 'no pain, no gain' passé?" *Journal of the American Medical Association*. Mar 21:285(11):1447-54.

50. Barclay, L., et. al. (2008) "Exercise may be needed to maintain weight loss in overweight women"; *Archives of Internal Medicine*. 168:1550-1559.

51. Cobb, K. (September 7, 2002) "Missed ZZZ's, More Disease?"; *Science News*. 162:152-154.

52. Gangwisch, JE., et. al. (2005) "Inadequate sleep as a risk factor for obesity: analysis of the NHANES I"; *Sleep*. 28(10):1289-1296.

53. Hellmich, N. (December 6, 2004) "Sleep loss may equal weight gain"; *USA Today*.

54. Spiegel, K., Van Cauter, E., et. al. (2004) "Brief communication: sleep curtailment in healthy young men is associated with decreased leptin levels, elevated ghrelin levels, and increased hunger and appetite"; *Annals of Internal Medicine*. Dec 7:141(11):846-50.

55. Spiegel, K. and Van Cauter, E., et. al. (1999) "Impact of sleep debt on metabolic and endocrine function"; *Lancet*. Oct 23:354(9188):1435-9

56. Gangwisch, JE., et. al. (2007) "Sleep duration as a risk factor for diabetes incidence in a large U.S. sample"; *Sleep*. December 1:30(12):1667–1673.

57. Cohen, S., et. al. (2009) "Sleep habits and susceptibility to the common cold"; *Archives of Internal Medicine*. 169(1):62-67.

58. Björntorp P. (1993) "Visceral obesity: a civilization syndrome"; *Obesity Research*. 1(3):206-22.

59. Blackburn, E. (2004) "Accelerated telomere shortening in response to life stress"; *PNAS*. December 7: Vol 101(49):17312-17315.

60. Ludlow, AT., et. al. (2008) "Relationship between physical activity level, telomere length, and telomerase activity"; *Medicine & Science in Sports & Exercise*. 40(10) October: 1764-1771.

61. Lewis, B., et.al. (2008) "The effect of exercise during pregnancy on maternal outcomes: practical implications for practice"; *American Journal of Lifestyle Medicine*. 2(5):441-455.

62. Clapp, JF. (2006) "Effects of diet and exercise on insulin resistance during pregnancy"; *Metabolic Syndrome and Related Disorders*. 4(2):84-90.

63. Clapp, JF. (2008) "Long-term outcome after exercising throughout pregnancy: fitness and cardiovascular risk"; *American Journal of Obstetrics and Gynecology*. 199(5):489e1-489e6.

64. Vliet, EL. (2001) *Women, weight and hormones: a weight loss plan for women over 35*. New York: M. Evans and Company, Inc.

65. Baillargeon, JP. (February 7, 2009) "Sex Hormones and Diabetes"; presented at the American Diabetes Association 56th Annual Postgraduate course.

66. Fried, SK., et. al. (1998) "Omental and subcutaneous adipose tissue of obese subjects release interleukin-6: depot difference and regulation by glucocorticoid"; *Journal of Clinical Endocrinology and Metabolism*. Mar:83(3):847-850.

67. Dokken, B. (2008) "The pathophysiology of cardiovascular disease and diabetes: beyond blood pressure and lipids"; *Diabetes Spectrum*. 21(3):160-165.

68. Bates, S., et. al. (March 2005) "Roles for leptin receptor/STAT3-dependent and independent signals in the regulation of glucose homeostasis"; *Cell Metabolism*. 1:169-178.

69. Myers, MG., et.al. (2005) "Leptin: a missing link between obesity and diabetes"; *Cell Metabolism*. 1(3):169-178.

70. Shapiro, A., et.al. (2008) "Fructose-induced leptin resistance exacerbates weight gain in response to subsequent high-fat feeding. Appetite, obesity and digestion"; *American Journal of Physiology - Regulatory, Integrative and Comparative Physiology*. 295:R1370-R1375.

71. O'Keefe, JH., et. al. (2008) "Dietary strategies for improving post-prandial glucose, lipids, inflammation, and cardiovascular health"; *Journal of American College of Cardiology*. 51(3).

72. Aroar, S., et. al. (2005) "The case for low carbohydrate diets in diabetes management"; *Nutrition and Metabolism*. 2:16-24.

73. Manninen, AH. (2004) "Is a calorie really a calorie? Metabolic advantage of low-carbohydrate diets"; *Journal of International Society of Sports Nutrition*. Dec 31:1(2):21-6.

74. Lane, JD., et. al. (2008) "Caffeine increases ambulatory glucose and postprandial responses in coffee drinkers with type 2 diabetes"; *Diabetes Care* 31:221-228.

75. Surwit, RS. (2004) *The Mind-Body Diabetes Revolution*. New York: Marlow and Company, pp. 220-221.

76. Fito, M., et. al. (2007) "Effect of a traditional Mediterranean diet on lipoprotein oxidation"; *Archives of Internal Medicine*. 167:1195-203.

77. Menato, G., et. al. (2008) "Current management of gestational diabetes mellitus"; *Expert Review of Obstetrics & Gynecology*. 3(1):73-91.

78. Nestler, J. (February 23, 2007) "Update on Polycystic Ovarian Syndrome"; Presented at the American Diabetes Association 54th Annual Postgraduate course.

79. The Rotterdam ESHRE/ASRM-sponsored PCOS consensus workshop group. "Revised 2003 consensus on diagnostic criteria and long-term health risks related to polycystic ovary syndrome"; (2004) *Human Reproduction*. 19:(1):41-47.

80. CDC, National Center for Health Statistics (April 11, 2008) www.cdc.gov.

81. Michaud, DS., et. al. (2002) "Dietary sugar, glycemic load, and pancreatic cancer risk in a prospective study"; *Journal of National Cancer Institute*. Sep 4:94(17):1293-1300.

82. Bergman, RN. (2003) "Insulin action and distribution of tissue blood flow"; *Journal of Clinical Endocrinology and Metabolism* 88(10):4556-4558.

83. Thompson, CL., et. al. (2008) "Carbohydrate consumption and esophageal cancer: an ecological assessment"; *The American Journal of Gastroenterology*. 103:555–561.

84. Ferrari, P., et. al. (2007) "Lifetime and baseline alcohol intake and risk of colon and rectal cancers in the European prospective investigation into cancer and nutrition"; *International Journal of Cancer*. 1:121(9):2065-2072.

85. Chen, WY. (2002) "Use of postmenopausal hormones, alcohol, and risk for invasive breast cancer"; *Annals of Internal Medicine*. 19 November:137(10):798-804.

86. Hatfield, J. (July/Aug/Sept 2005) "Exercise and Nutritional strategies for breast cancer prevention"; *ACSM News*. 15(3):8-10.

87. Allen, NE., et al. (2009) "Moderate Alcohol Intake and Cancer Incidence in Women"; *Journal of the National Cancer Institute*. 101(5):296-305.

88. Chobanian AV., et. al. (2003) "Blood pressure: The JNC report"; *Journal of the American Medical Association*. 289:2560-2572.

89. Fung, TT., et. al. (April 14, 2008) "Adherence to a DASH-style diet and risk of coronary heart disease and stoke in woman"; *Archives of Internal Medicine*. 168:713-720.

90. Wildman, RP., et. al. (August 11, 2008) "The obese without cardiometabolic risk factor clustering and the normal weight with cardiometabolic risk factor clustering: prevalence of correlates of 2 phenotypes among the U.S. population" (NHANES 1999-2004). *Archives of Internal Medicine*. 168(15): 45:1617-24.

91. Isoldi, KK., et. al. (2008) "The challenge of treating obesity: the endocannabiniod system as a potential target"; *Journal of the American Dietetics Association*. 108:823-831.

92. Kritchevsky, SB. (2004) "A review of scientific research and recommendations regarding eggs"; *Journal of the American College of Nutrition*. 23(6 suppl):596S-600S.

93. Hu, FB., et. al. (1999) "A prospective study of egg consumption and risk of cardiovascular disease in men and women"; *Journal of the American Medical Association*. 281:1387-1394

94. Qureshi AL., et. al. (2007) "Regular egg consumption does not increase the risk of stroke and cardiovascular disease"; *Medical Science Monitor*. Jan:13(1):CR1-8.

95. Djousse, E., and Gaziano, JM. (April

2008) "Egg consumption in relation to cardiovascular disease and mortality: the Physician's Health Study"; *American Journal of Clinical Nutrition.* 87(4):964-969.

96. Gray, J., and Griffin, B. (March 209) "Eggs and dietary cholesterol – dispelling the myth"; *Nutrition Bulletin.* 34:66-70.

97. Kremer, JM. (2000) "Omega-3 fatty acid supplements in rheumatoid arthritis"; *American Journal of Clinical Nutrition.* 71:349S-351S.

98. Giovannucci, E., et. al. (2007) "Can vitamin D reduce total mortality?"; *Archives of Internal Medicine.* 167:1709-1710, 1730-1737.

99. Vemulapalli, R. (2008) "Diet and lifestyle modifications in the management of gastroesophageal reflux disease"; *Nutrition in Clinical Practice.* Jun-Jul:23(3):293-8.

100. Fava, M. (2000) "Weight gain and antidepressants"; *Journal of Clinical Psychiatry.* 61(supp 11):37-41.

101. Deshmukh, R., et. al. (July 2003) "Managing weight gain as a side effect of antidepressant therapy"; *Cleveland Journal of Medicine.* 70(7):614-623.

102. Lasslo-Meeks, M. (Spring 2003) "Weight gain of psychotropic and seizure disorder medications"; *SCAN's Pulse.* p. 7-12.

103. Wofford, MR., et. al. (2004) "Relationship between antihypertensive drugs and metabolic syndrome"; *Metabolic Syndrome of Related Disorders.* Fall:2(4):308 14.

Index